Tim Kreutzmann

Geometric Regularization in Bioluminescence Tomography

Geometric Regularization in Bioluminescence Tomography

by
Tim Kreutzmann

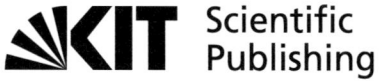

Dissertation, Karlsruher Institut für Technologie (KIT)
Fakultät für Mathematik, 2013
Tag der mündlichen Prüfung: 13. November 2013

Impressum

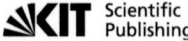 Scientific
Publishing

Karlsruher Institut für Technologie (KIT)
KIT Scientific Publishing
Straße am Forum 2
D-76131 Karlsruhe

KIT Scientific Publishing is a registered trademark of Karlsruhe
Institute of Technology. Reprint using the book cover is not allowed.

www.ksp.kit.edu

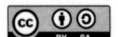
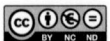
Print on Demand 2014

ISBN 978-3-7315 -0142-8

Geometric Regularization in Bioluminescence Tomography

Zur Erlangung des akademischen Grades eines

DOKTORS DER NATURWISSENSCHAFTEN

von der Fakultät für Mathematik des
Karlsruher Instituts für Technologie (KIT)
genehmigte

DISSERTATION

von

Dipl.-Math. techn. Tim Kreutzmann
aus Groß-Gerau

Tag der mündlichen Prüfung: 13. November 2013
Referent: Prof. Dr. Andreas Rieder
Korreferent: PD Dr. Frank Hettlich

Contents

CHAPTER 1

Introduction

Bioluminescence tomography (BLT) is a novel biomedical imaging technique to study molecular and cellular activities in a living organism noninvasively. The method is based on bioluminescence imaging (BLI), whose potential is described by Dr. David Piwnica-Worms in [**Ban05**]: *"It can be applied to all disease processes in all areas of small-animal models."*

As the name suggests, the underlying phenomenon is bioluminescence, which is the capability of an organism to emit light. Well-known examples of animals with these genetic endowments are fireflies or jellyfishes. The light emission is due to an oxidation of a substrate, the so-called luciferin, under the presence of an enzyme, the luciferase, which is encoded by the DNA of the organism.

The idea of bioluminescence imaging is the tagging of target cells, e.g. tumor cells, by the luciferase gene. When the luciferin is then injected prior to imaging, the tagged cells emit light and the photons exiting the organism are recorded by a sensitive camera. In Figure 1.1 typical bioluminescence imaging data are shown. Since the tag is encoded in the genes, the intensity of the signal of a cell is not reduced after cell division. Thus, bioluminescence imaging is suitable for *in vivo* studies over a long period of time. In addition, it is a very sensitive method with a high signal-to-noise ratio, as no external light source is required. Besides the capability of bioluminescence imaging to track the tagged cells, it also allows to image biological events using engineered luciferase. Thus, it serves

1

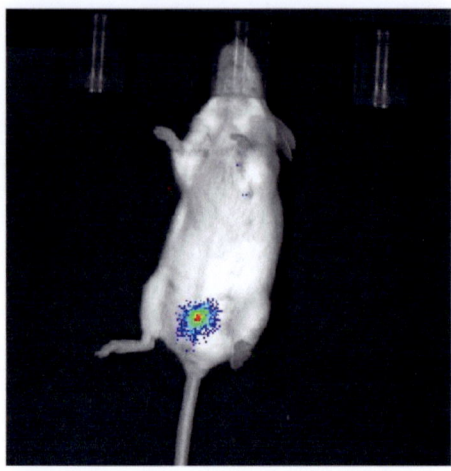

FIGURE 1.1. Bioluminescence imaging data by courtesy of Dr. Mustafa Diken, In Vivo Imaging Core Facility, TRON – Translational Oncology at the University Medical Center Mainz.

"as an eyepiece into biology" [**CR02**]. However, due to absorption of light in animal tissue, bioluminescence imaging is limited to depths of a few centimeters. In view of this fact together with the inherent infiltration of genes into the target cells, it becomes clear that the main application of bioluminescence imaging is in preclinical studies using small animal models. For a more detailed discussion of bioluminescence imaging we refer to [**Ban05, CR02, TC05, WN03**]; see also [**Kre08**].

As a planar imaging technique, bioluminescence imaging suffers from the structural drawback that it gives only two-dimensional information on the bioluminescent source. To overcome this limitation, mathematics comes into play. Given the exiting photons over the whole surface of the organism and a model describing the propagation of light in tissue, the problem of bioluminescence tomography is to find the three-dimensional location and intensity of the bioluminescent source.

This problem belongs to the class of inverse problems, cf. [**Isa06, Kir11, Rie03**], since the effect, the exiting photons over the organism's surface, is known and the cause, the light source, is sought. More precisely, the bioluminescence tomography problem is an interior source problem. As many inverse problems in science, it is ill-posed: small perturbations of the measurements can lead to large errors in the reconstruction.

For the description of light propagation in tissue, needed in the reconstruction process of bioluminescence tomography, two models are essentially used in practice. *"The most comprehensive model"* [**NW01**] is the transport model where the photon flux is described by the radiative transfer equation, an integro-differential equation depending on a spatial and an angular variable. In scattering media, like animal tissue, the diffusion model is a good approximation to the transport model. It is based on the diffusion equation, also called diffusion approximation, a second-order elliptic partial differential equation over the spatial domain. The former model is rather complex, whereas the latter is simpler. Both models require knowledge of the optical properties of the object to be imaged. This information is usually obtained by a prior X-ray computed tomography (CT) or magnetic resonance imaging (MRI) scan.

In the early years after the patent application in 2003 [**WHM**] the diffusion approximation and the classical Tikhonov regularization scheme were mostly used as the mathematical model and the reconstruction method, respectively, cf. [**HCW06a, WCD$^+$06, WCL$^+$06**]. We point out that the latter two articles particularly give a description of the BLT system design. However, other reconstruction methods were also applied, e.g. a (unregularized) Newton method in [**CWK$^+$05**] and a Levenberg–Marquardt method in [**GZLJ04**]. Questions on uniqueness of the BLT problem are addressed in [**WLJ04**]. In the following years extensions of the BLT problem based on Tikhonov regularization and the diffusion model were developed: multispectral bioluminescence tomography [**HCW06b, HW07, JW08**], bioluminescence tomography with a simultaneous adjustment of the optical parameters [**HKCW07**] and with a simultaneous reconstruction of the optical parameters [**HCKW09, HGC13**], temperature-modulated bioluminescence tomography [**HSK$^+$09**] and bioluminescence tomography for media with spatially varying refractive index [**GCH10**]. A summary of the early extensions can be found in the review article [**HW08**]. For a further analysis of the finite element method applied to the BLT problem, besides the one presented in [**HCW06a**], we refer to [**GLYZ08, GC13**]. In the last few years two new trends appeared in the area of bioluminescence tomography, namely using the transport model and sparse reconstruction methods. Schemes involving an l^1 regularization term of the discretized source based on the diffusion model and the transport model are proposed in [**LZD$^+$09**] and [**GZ10a**], respectively. Latter approach is extended in [**GZ10b**] to an l^1 plus total variation (TV) regularization method incorporating either an l^1 or an l^2 residual. The BLT problem based on the transport model and using the classical Tikhonov

regularization is analyzed in [**HEHL11**]. In [**Ben11, ZLC12**] a Poisson
noise model for the BLT problem based on the diffusion approximation is
considered and appropriate reconstruction schemes are developed, where
the data misfit is measured with the Kullback–Leibler divergence and an
l^1 or l^0 regularization term is used.[1]

Although many different approaches for bioluminescence tomography
have been proposed in the last ten years, none of them has prevailed in
practice. Consequently, further research is needed in order to find a reliable
reconstruction method that will become widely accepted.

In this work we investigate a novel approach for bioluminescence tomography. The basis for this approach is the *a priori* knowledge that
the source is a piecewise constant function, which is due to the nature
of the bioluminescent source given by tagged cells. Rather than search-
ing for an arbitrary source function, we aim to reconstruct the support of
the source and the corresponding intensity. To face the ill-posedness of
the BLT problem, we stabilize the reconstruction process by a Tikhonov
like functional with a perimeter penalty term. This choice is inspired by
[**RR07**], where this stability term is used in the CT framework, and by
[**GZ10b**], where TV regularization for the BLT problem is incorporated.
This leads to our *geometric regularization approach for bioluminescence
tomography* based on both models, the radiative transfer equation and the
diffusion approximation.

For the regularized problem, a minimization problem over the nonlinear and non-convex set of shapes, we develop positive answers to fundamental questions: existence of a solution, stability and regularization
property. An approximate variational principle is shown, which ensures the
existence of smooth almost stationary shapes near the minimizer. These
findings build the first key contribution of this thesis. These results in the
diffusion based framework were published in [**KR12**].

To solve the minimization problem, shape optimization methods involving the domain derivative of the Tikhonov like functional are applied.
In contrast to the diffusion model, where the domain derivative of the forward operator is known from the derivation in [**Het99**], the rigorous calculation of the domain derivative of the forward operator in the transport
model is a challenging task. To our knowledge, it has not been performed
before. We rigorously derive the domain derivative about ball-shaped

---

[1]For the sake of completeness, we note that in nearly all of the mentioned papers
a priori knowledge on the source, like non-negativity or a permissible region for the
support, is implemented by constraining the respective optimization problem.

sources in the transport model. This forms the second key contribution of this thesis.

As always in mathematics, the results of this work are not restricted to the specific application of bioluminescence tomography, but also hold for application with a similar mathematical structure. For instance, the inverse gravimetry problem [**Isa06**] is similar to the BLT problem based on the diffusion model; single photon emission computed tomography (SPECT) [**NW01**] is a special case of bioluminescence tomography based on the transport model, namely the special case without scattering. Furthermore, the BLT problem is closely related to the inverse source problem occurring in fluorescence tomography [**EFS10, KNH05**].

This thesis is structured into four parts. In Part I the general framework covering both models is treated. In Chapter 2 the transport model is motivated and the diffusion model is derived from it. Then, the Tikhonov like functional is introduced and the regularized problem under investigation is formulated. Chapter 3 contains an analytical discussion of the regularized problem: existence, stability and regularization property as well as an approximate variational principle are developed. This discussion is followed by a self-contained theory for star-shaped domains giving analogous results.

In Part II the BLT problem based on the diffusion approximation is further investigated. The domain derivative of the corresponding forward operator is derived in Chapter 4 and consequences for the regularized problem are deduced. In Chapter 5 numerical schemes based on the theoretical findings are proposed and tested for star-shaped sources in two dimensions.

The BLT problem based on the radiative transfer equation is addressed in Part III. In Chapter 6 the domain differentiability of the forward operator in the transport framework is discussed and rigorously derived about ball-shaped sources. Consequences for the regularized problem follow. The theoretical results and heuristic generalizations are numerically verified in Chapter 7, wherein all experiments are performed on star-shaped sources in three dimensions.

Chapter 8 gives a short summary and an outlook on future research.

In the Appendices, which build the fourth part, supplementary results are presented in order to complete this thesis. Particularly, we point out Appendix D and Appendix E, where the singular value decomposition of the BLT forward operator based on the diffusion model and the domain derivative of the SPECT forward operator are derived.

Before we get started on the detailed discussion, I want to thank several people for their support while writing this thesis. First and foremost,

I am deeply grateful to my advisor Prof. Dr. Andreas Rieder. He has provided constant encouragement and friendly guidance through all stages of my thesis. I thank my co-advisor PD Dr. Frank Hettlich for fruitful discussions and his inputs, particularly on the domain derivative. I thank Prof. Dr. Weimin Han (The University of Iowa) for the opportunity to research in his working group for six months. This exchange has had many positive effects on my work. The visit was partly funded by the Karlsruhe House of Young Scientists (KHYS), whose support is greatly acknowledged. I give special thanks to Dr. Joseph Eichholz (Rose-Hulman Institute of Technology) for providing RTEPACK and implementing a few extensions used in this work. I am grateful to my former student assistants Christian Wegend and Ekaterina Kovacheva for doing some of the technical coding. Many thanks go to my colleagues at Karlsruhe and Iowa for the stimulating conversations and the very nice atmosphere. Among my colleagues, I am particularly grateful to Prof. Dr. Andreas Kirsch, who introduced me to the field of inverse problems back in my student years, and to Fábio Margotti, Dr. Daniel Maurer, Dr. Vikram Sunkara and Robert Winkler for their inputs improving this thesis. Finally, I cannot thank my entire family enough for their endless support.

Part I
General Framework

CHAPTER 2

Problem Statement

In this chapter we introduce the problem under investigation in this thesis. We start by presenting two models of light propagation in tissue, the transport model based on the radiative transfer equation (RTE) and the diffusion model based on the diffusion approximation (DA). Former is the *"most comprehensive model"* [**NW01**], but in scattering media latter is a good approximation reducing the computational costs. Given the description of light transport in tissue, we can formulate the inverse source problem of bioluminescence tomography. As this problem is ill-posed, *a priori* knowledge on the source term and a penalty term is used to stabilize the reconstruction process. This results in a minimization problem of a Tikhonov like functional, sometimes also called Mumford–Shah like functional.

2.1. Mathematical Models of Light Propagation in Tissue

The presentation in this section is based on Chapter 2 of [**Kre08**] and the literature mentioned there, namely [**Arr02, BGCC99, NW01**], as well as [**CZ67**]. For the sake of completeness, the derivation of the two models is recalled here.

2.1.1. The Transport Model. Let $d \in \{2,3\}$ and $X \subset \mathbb{R}^d$ be the spatial domain, i.e., the object of interest. The propagation of light in this object consisting of animal tissue follows the laws of particle transport [**Arr02**]. To be more precise, we consider the photon flux $u = u(x,\omega,t)$, which is the energy density or equivalently the density of photons in the point $x \in X$ traveling into direction $\omega \in \Omega$ at time t. Herein, Ω is the $(d-1)$-dimensional unit sphere S^{d-1}, the angular domain. The change of the photon flux in time is the sum of the physical phenomena emission, absorption, scattering and propagation. In other words, the time derivative $\frac{\partial}{\partial t}u$ satisfies the balance relation, cf. [**BGCC99, CZ67**]:

$$\frac{\partial u}{\partial t} = \left[\frac{\partial u}{\partial t}\right]_{\text{em}} + \left[\frac{\partial u}{\partial t}\right]_{\text{abs}} + \left[\frac{\partial u}{\partial t}\right]_{\text{scat}} + \left[\frac{\partial u}{\partial t}\right]_{\text{prop}} . \qquad (2.1)$$

The first summand in (2.1), evaluated at (x, ω, t), describes photons that are emitted in the spatial point x in the direction ω at time t. It can be written as

$$\left[\frac{\partial u}{\partial t}\right]_{\text{em}} (x, \omega, t) = cq(x, \omega, t),$$

where q is the source term and c the constant photon speed.

The second term in (2.1) models the absorption of photons, which is proportional to the photon flux. Introducing the space dependent[1] absorption coefficient σ_{a}, we have

$$\left[\frac{\partial u}{\partial t}\right]_{\text{abs}} (x, \omega, t) = -c\sigma_{\text{a}}(x)u(x, \omega, t).$$

The scattering term consists of two parts,

$$\left[\frac{\partial u}{\partial t}\right]_{\text{scat}} = \left[\frac{\partial u}{\partial t}\right]_{\text{out}} + \left[\frac{\partial u}{\partial t}\right]_{\text{in}} .$$

First, photons coming from the direction ω are scattered into a different direction ω'. This phenomenon is like absorption proportional to the photon flux u and thus

$$\left[\frac{\partial u}{\partial t}\right]_{\text{out}} (x, \omega, t) = -c\sigma_{\text{s}}(x)u(x, \omega, t)$$

holds with the scattering coefficient σ_{s}. Second, photons coming from a different direction ω' are scattered into the direction ω. To describe this phenomenon, we introduce the scattering kernel η, depending on the spatial variable x and the angle $\omega \cdot \omega'$, that represents the probability of

---

[1]We point out explicitly that in the general theory the absorption coefficient as well as the scattering coefficient and kernel might depend on the angular variable ω. But in optical tomography, it is a standard assumption that these quantities are angularly independent, see e.g. [**Arr02, NW01**].

a photon coming from direction ω' being scattered into direction ω under the condition that this photon is scattered. It is normalized such that

$$\int_\Omega \eta(x, \omega \cdot \omega') \, d\omega' = 1 . \tag{2.2}$$

In view of the first part modeling the condition that a photon is scattered, we obtain

$$\left[\frac{\partial u}{\partial t}\right]_{\text{in}} (x, \omega, t) = c\sigma_{\text{s}}(x) \int_\Omega \eta(x, \omega \cdot \omega') u(x, \omega', t) \, d\omega' .$$

The last summand in (2.1) characterizes photons traveling without changes in direction and corresponds to the directional derivative, that is,

$$\left[\frac{\partial u}{\partial t}\right]_{\text{prop}} (x, \omega, t) = -c\omega \cdot \nabla_x u(x, \omega, t) .$$

Using the characterizations of the summands of (2.1), we obtain that the photon flux u satisfies the time-dependent radiative transfer equation

$$\frac{1}{c}\frac{\partial u}{\partial t}(x, \omega, t) + \omega \cdot \nabla_x u(x, \omega, t) + \sigma_{\text{t}}(x) u(x, \omega, t)$$
$$= \sigma_{\text{s}}(x) \int_\Omega \eta(x, \omega \cdot \omega') u(x, \omega', t) \, d\omega' + q(x, \omega, t) \tag{2.3}$$

with the total attenuation coefficient $\sigma_{\text{t}} = \sigma_{\text{a}} + \sigma_{\text{s}}$.

In addition to the behavior inside the object, we have to model the boundary conditions, i.e., photons entering and leaving the domain X. The sets

$$\partial_{\mp}(X \times \Omega) = \{(x, \omega) \in \partial X \times \Omega : \omega \cdot \nu(x) \lessgtr 0\}$$

are called inflow and outflow part of the boundary $\partial X \times \Omega$, respectively. Herein, ν is the outer unit normal to X. Depending on the environment the experiments are performed in, a function g^- defined on the inflow boundary describes the incoming photons, that is,

$$u(x, \omega, t) = g^-(x, \omega, t) \quad \text{for } (x, \omega) \in \partial_-(X \times \Omega) .$$

In an ideal setting the measurements are taken on the whole outflow boundary and are angularly resolved, that is, we measure the function

$$g(x, \omega, t) = u(x, \omega, t) \quad \text{for } (x, \omega) \in \partial_+(X \times \Omega) .$$

Despite the fact that in practice it is often only possible to measure angularly averaged [**Bal09**], i.e.,

$$\int_{\Omega_{x,+}} u(x, \omega, t)\nu(x) \cdot \omega \, d\omega \quad \text{for } x \in \partial X$$

with

$$\Omega_{x,\pm} = \left\{ \omega \in \Omega \colon \omega \cdot \nu(x) \gtrless 0 \right\},$$

we will assume angularly resolved data in this thesis. This choice is discussed below.

In the above derivation of the radiative transfer equation and the boundary conditions we considered the time-dependent case for the sake of presentation. However, in bioluminescence tomography the photon source q induced by reporter genes is relatively stable over time [**NRWW05, WLJ04**] and thus we change over to the stationary case. Moreover, we assume that the source is isotropic, i.e., independent of ω. This is reasonable knowing that the source is built up of marked cells; it is also a standard assumption in RTE-based BLT, cf. [**GZ10a, HEHL11**]. Since the measurements are usually taken in a dark environment, we restrict ourselves to homogeneous inflow boundary conditions.

With the definition of the scattering operator

$$(Su)(x,\omega) = \sigma_{\mathrm{s}}(x) \int_{\Omega} \eta(x, \omega \cdot \omega') u(x, \omega') \, \mathrm{d}\omega' \qquad (2.4)$$

we finally obtain the stationary radiative transfer equation in the form

$$\omega \cdot \nabla_x u(x,\omega) + \sigma_{\mathrm{t}}(x) u(x,\omega) - Su(x,\omega) = q(x) \quad \text{for } (x,\omega) \in X \times \Omega \quad (2.5)$$

and the homogeneous inflow boundary conditions

$$u(x,\omega) = 0 \quad \text{for } (x,\omega) \in \partial_-(X \times \Omega). \qquad (2.6)$$

In view of the time-independence of the photon flux u, the measurements are independent as well and given by

$$g(x,\omega) = u(x,\omega) \quad \text{for } (x,\omega) \in \partial_+(X \times \Omega). \qquad (2.7)$$

The last three equations build our model of RTE-based BLT in this work. To be more precise, when we speak of the RTE-based BLT problem, we refer to the problem of finding the source function q such that the solution u of the boundary value problem (2.5)–(2.6) meets the measurements (2.7).

With the final form of the RTE model complete, we return to the discussion of the choice of measurements. Though in practice angularly resolved measurements are hard to obtain, these are the measurements to aim for. In case of angular averaging we have to reconstruct the source function q over a d-dimensional domain given data over a $(d-1)$-dimensional manifold. This lack of information in one dimension leads to

non-uniqueness of the BLT problem and worsens the ill-posedness.[2] For
the applications this means that we only get unreliable reconstructions.
Therefore, we restrict ourselves to the angularly resolved framework and
expect that future technology makes these kind of measurements possible
in practice.

We point out that we have not treated the case of photons leaving and
re-entering the domain X explicitly yet. Implicitly we assumed that this
effect does not occur, as the chosen boundary conditions do not allow this
event. Therefore, we assume either that X is convex or that the measure
geometry prevents re-entrance of photons, e.g. in the idealistic setup where
the measurements are taken directly on the boundary.

One drawback of the transport model is that the solution of the radiative transfer equation depends on $2d - 1$ variables, thus solving this
is computational costly. Therefore, we derive in the next section a simpler model that is a good description of light propagation in tissue if the
predominant phenomenon is scattering rather than transport [**AS09**].

2.1.2. The Diffusion Model. In bioluminescence tomography the
scattering length σ_s^{-1} and thus also the free mean path between inter-
actions σ_t^{-1} are typically small compared to the object size. In [**Arr02**]
it is mentioned that typical values for the coefficients in tissue are $\sigma_a =
0.01 - 0.1$ mm^{-1} and $\sigma_s = 10 - 20$ mm^{-1}. By contrast, [**NW01**] refer
to $\sigma_s = 100 - 200$ mm^{-1} as typical values for the scattering coefficient.
The object under observation is usually a mouse and thus the diameter
and length are of a larger order of magnitude than the scattering length.
Therefore, the predominant phenomenon is scattering and the photon flux
is essentially isotropic a small distance away from the source. Hence, we
assume that the photon flux u depends only linearly on ω.

To specify this assumption, we introduce the first moments of u:

$$u_0(x) = \frac{1}{\mathrm{Vol}(\Omega)} \int_\Omega u(x,\omega) \, \mathrm{d}\omega \in \mathbb{R} \,,$$

$$u_1(x) = \frac{1}{\mathrm{Vol}(\Omega)} \int_\Omega \omega u(x,\omega) \, \mathrm{d}\omega \in \mathbb{R}^d \,,$$

$$u_2(x) = \frac{1}{\mathrm{Vol}(\Omega)} \int_\Omega \omega \omega^T u(x,\omega) \, \mathrm{d}\omega \in \mathbb{R}^{d \times d} \,.$$

---

[2]In Section 2.2.2 and Part II of this thesis, where the DA-based BLT problem is
discussed, the effect of the lack of information becomes apparent. Though the model
is different there, the dimension of the data is also one less than the dimension of the
source to be reconstructed.

The quantity $\text{Vol}(\Omega)u_0(x)$ describes the density of photons in the point x and is therefore known as photon density.

We remark that we still consider the stationary case and assume that q is isotropic. The derivation of the diffusion approximation in the time-dependent case and with an anisotropic source can be found in [**Arr02**] or [**Kre08**]. Moreover, we restrict ourselves in this subsection to the case $d = 3$. The derivation of the diffusion model for $d = 2$ is postponed to the Appendix B.2, as the derivation is identical in principle, only a few constants differ.

Let us now make the crucial assumption that u only depends linearly on ω, i.e.,

$$u(x, \omega) = a(x) + b(x) \cdot \omega \qquad (2.8)$$

with a real-valued function a and a function b with values in $\mathbb{R}^3$. We obtain these two functions by inserting the ansatz (2.8) in the definition of the moments u_0 and u_1:

$$a(x) = u_0(x) \quad \text{and} \quad b(x) = 3u_1(x).$$

Herein, we used the identities (B.1) and (B.2) of the appendix

$$\int_\Omega \omega \, d\omega = 0 \quad \text{and} \quad \int_\Omega \omega\omega^T \, d\omega = \frac{4\pi}{3} I.$$

Consequently, u obeys the form

$$u(x, \omega) = u_0(x) + 3u_1(x) \cdot \omega. \qquad (2.9)$$

Furthermore, we can apply the Funk–Hecke formula (A.4) to the scattering kernel and observe

$$\int_\Omega \omega' \eta(x, \omega \cdot \omega') \, d\omega' = \overline{\eta_1}(x)\omega \qquad (2.10)$$

with

$$\overline{\eta_1}(x) = 4\pi \int_{-1}^{1} \eta(x, t)t \, dt.$$

Now we have all quantities needed at hand and can derive the diffusion approximation from the radiative transfer equation. Integration of latter, i.e., equation (2.5), over Ω leads to

$$\nabla \cdot u_1(x) + \sigma_a(x)u_0(x) = q(x), \qquad (2.11)$$

where we used the normalization (2.2) of η. Multiplying the radiative transfer equation (2.5) by ω and then integrating over Ω, we obtain

$$(\nabla \cdot u_2(x))^T + \sigma_t(x)u_1(x) - \overline{\eta_1}(x)\sigma_s(x)u_1(x) = 0. \qquad (2.12)$$

To clarify the last step, we recall (2.10) as well as (B.1), i.e., $\int_\Omega \omega \, d\omega = 0$.

The next step is to eliminate the term u_2 from (2.12). Inserting the form of u (2.9) in the definition of u_2, we observe the relation

$$(\nabla \cdot u_2)^T = \frac{1}{3}\nabla u_0 \,,$$

since

$$\int_\Omega \omega\omega^T \, d\omega = \frac{4\pi}{3}I \quad \text{and} \quad \int_\Omega (\omega \cdot a)\omega\omega^T \, d\omega = 0 \,.$$

Both integrals are calculated in Appendix B.1, compare equations (B.2) and (B.3). Thus, we are able to eliminate u_2 and the equations (2.11) and (2.12) become the following system of differential equations:

$$\nabla \cdot u_1 + \sigma_\mathrm{a}u_0 = q \,,$$
$$\frac{1}{3}\nabla u_0 + (\sigma_\mathrm{a} + \sigma'_\mathrm{s})u_1 = 0 \tag{2.13}$$

with the reduced scattering coefficient $\sigma'_\mathrm{s} = (1 - \overline{\eta_1})\sigma_s$. From the second equation in (2.13) follows immediately that

$$u_1 = -D\nabla u_0 \quad \text{with} \quad D = \frac{1}{3(\sigma_\mathrm{a} + \sigma'_\mathrm{s})} \,. \tag{2.14}$$

The factor D is called diffusion coefficient. The use of the last relation in the first equation of (2.13) finally yields the diffusion approximation

$$-\nabla \cdot \big(D\nabla u_0\big) + \sigma_\mathrm{a}u_0 = q \quad \text{in } X \,. \tag{2.15}$$

Sometimes we will also refer to this differential equation as diffusion equation.

In order to complete the diffusion model, we transfer the boundary conditions. Integrating the homogeneous inflow boundary conditions (2.6) weighted by $\nu \cdot \omega$ over the inward pointing directions, we obtain

$$\int_{\nu(x)\cdot\omega<0} \nu(x) \cdot \omega u(x,\omega) \, d\omega = 0 \quad \text{for } x \in \partial X \,.$$

For the simplification of the left-hand side we observe that

$$\int_{\nu\cdot\omega<0} \nu \cdot \omega \, d\omega = -\pi \quad \text{and} \quad \int_{\nu\cdot\omega<0} (\nu \cdot \omega)\omega \, d\omega = \frac{2\pi}{3}\nu$$

for $\nu \in \Omega$. These integrals are derived in the appendix, cf. (B.4). Now we write u in the form (2.9) and use the identity (2.14) to deduce the Robin boundary condition

$$u_0 + 2D\frac{\partial u_0}{\partial \nu} = 0 \quad \text{on } \partial X \,. \tag{2.16}$$

The measurement in the diffusion model is the angularly averaged outflow, i.e., the weighted integral of (2.7) over the outward pointing directions,

$$g_0(x) = \int_{\nu(x)\cdot\omega>0} \nu(x)\cdot\omega u(x,\omega)\,\mathrm{d}\omega \quad \text{for } x \in \partial X\,.$$

In view of the homogeneous inflow boundary condition (2.6), the definition of u_1 as well as the formula (2.14), the measurements can be rewritten as

$$g_0(x) = \nu(x)\cdot u_1(x) = -D(x)\nu(x)\cdot\nabla u_0(x) \quad \text{for } x \in \partial X\,,$$

which is nothing other than the Neumann boundary condition

$$D\frac{\partial u_0}{\partial \nu} = -g_0 \quad \text{on } \partial X\,. \tag{2.17}$$

The equations (2.15)–(2.17) form the diffusion model of bioluminescence tomography. The DA-based BLT problem is to find the source function q such that the solution u_0 of the boundary value problem (2.15)–(2.16) satisfies the measurements (2.17).

Let us shortly and for the last time in this thesis come back to the two-dimensional diffusion approximation. As we derive in Appendix B.2, the photon density with no incoming photons is described by the boundary value problem

$$-\nabla\cdot\left(D\nabla u_0\right) + \sigma_a u_0 = q \quad \text{in } X\,,$$

$$u_0 + \frac{\pi}{2}D\frac{\partial u_0}{\partial \nu} = 0 \quad \text{on } \partial X$$

with the adapted diffusion coefficient

$$D = \frac{1}{2(\sigma_a + \sigma_s')}\,.$$

This adaption is also the only change in the measurements, which are

$$D\frac{\partial u_0}{\partial \nu} = -g_0 \quad \text{on } \partial X\,.$$

We observe, this is also mentioned before, that the only difference are the coefficients in the differential equation and in the boundary condition. However, the type of the differential equation and boundary condition remains the same and thus the properties of the direct and also inverse problem are conserved. For the ease of presentation, we will only consider the three-dimensional diffusion model, i.e., equations (2.15), (2.16) and (2.17), independent of the value of d, though we are aware that for $d = 2$ the transferred model has different coefficients. In fact, the case $d = 3$ is the case occurring in practice.

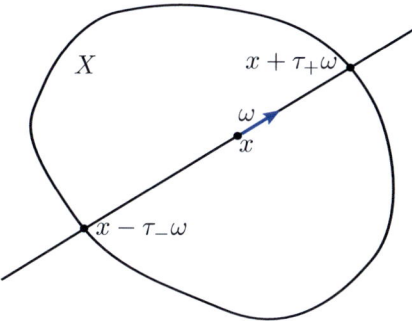

FIGURE 2.1. Sketch of the geometry and time of travel.

2.2. Bioluminescence Tomography Problem

Based on the developed models of photon propagation in tissue, we now want to analyze the problem of bioluminescence tomography in more detail. We recall the problem statement: Given the measurements g in the transport model or g_0 in the diffusion model, find the source function q such that the equations (2.5)–(2.7) or (2.15)–(2.17) are satisfied, respectively.

In the following we formalize this problem for each model separately and sketch the ill-posedness. These insights build the foundation and motivation to the regularization scheme introduced in the next section.

2.2.1. RTE-based BLT Problem. Let us begin by stating the assumptions on the domain and the coefficients in order to obtain a well-posed direct problem. When working in the transport setting and not mentioned otherwise, we assume that X is a bounded domain with sufficiently smooth boundary (at least Lipschitz continuous) and that the coefficients σ_t, σ_s are non-negative and in $L^\infty(X)$ as well as that the kernel η is also non-negative and satisfies the normalization condition (2.2), i.e.,

$$\int_\Omega \eta(x, \omega \cdot \omega') \, d\omega' = 1 \quad \text{for a.e. } (x, \omega) \in X \times \Omega.$$

Additionally, we assume the subcritical situation: There exists a positive constant σ_0 such that

$$\sigma_a = \sigma_t - \sigma_s \geq \sigma_0 > 0 \quad \text{a.e. on } X. \tag{2.18}$$

Next we introduce the function spaces we work in and present important properties of them. For $p \in [1, \infty]$ let $L^p(X \times \Omega)$ be the usual

Lebesgue spaces on the manifold $X \times \Omega$ and

$$W^p = W^p(X \times \Omega) = \{v \in L^p(X \times \Omega) \colon \omega \cdot \nabla v \in L^p(X \times \Omega)\},$$
$$W^p_- = W^p_-(X \times \Omega) = \{v \in W^p(X \times \Omega) \colon v|_{\partial_-(X \times \Omega)} = 0\}.$$

We point out soon how to understand the trace condition $v|_{\partial_-(X \times \Omega)} = 0$ in the latter definition. Both spaces, W^p and W^p_-, equipped with the norm

$$\|v\|_{W^p} = \|v\|_{L^p} + \|\omega \cdot \nabla v\|_{L^p}$$

are Banach spaces. For $p \in [1, \infty[$ the space $C^\infty(\overline{X} \times \Omega)$ is dense in $W^p(X \times \Omega)$ [**DL00b**]. Moreover, we know from [**DL00b**, Chapter XXI, §2.1] that for $v \in W^p(X \times \Omega)$, $p \in [1, \infty]$, the identity

$$\frac{\partial}{\partial t} v(x + t\omega, \omega)\Big|_{t=0} = \omega \cdot \nabla v(x, \omega) \tag{2.19}$$

holds for almost all $(x, \omega) \in X \times \Omega$, where all derivatives are understood in the weak sense.

For functions in $L^1(X \times \Omega)$ there is a standard change of variables result. To formulate it, the time of travel is needed, which is defined by

$$\tau_\pm(x, \omega) = \sup\{t \colon x \pm s\omega \in X \text{ for } 0 \leq s < t\} \quad \text{for } (x, \omega) \in X \times \Omega.$$

For an illustration of the time of travel we refer to Figure 2.1. The change of variables result, which is adopted from [**CS99**, Lemma 2.1], is now the following lemma:

Lemma 2.1. *For $u \in L^1(X \times \Omega)$ holds*

$$\int_\Omega \int_X u(x, \omega) \, \mathrm{d}x \, \mathrm{d}\omega = \int_\Omega \int_{\partial X_{\omega, \mp}} \int_0^{\tau_\pm(y, \omega)} u(y \pm t\omega, \omega) |\omega \cdot \nu(y)| \, \mathrm{d}t \, \mathrm{d}\mu(y) \, \mathrm{d}\omega$$

with $\partial X_{\omega, \mp} = \{x \in \partial X \colon \nu(x) \cdot \omega \lessgtr 0\}$ and $\mathrm{d}\mu$ the surface measure on ∂X.

This Lemma is used to prove the following trace theorems. The idea to show these is to apply the mean value theorem on each line $\{y - t\omega \colon t \in [0, \bar{t}]\}$ for $\bar{t} \leq \tau_-(y, \omega)$ and $(y, \omega) \in \partial_+(X \times \Omega)$ and to use this to estimate $|v(y, \omega)|$. If $p = \infty$, the statement is an easy observation. In case $p \in [1, \infty[$, integration of this estimate together with Lemma 2.1 yields the next two statements. The detailed proofs can be found in [**Ces84, Ces85**].

Lemma 2.2. *Let $c > 0$ be an arbitrary constant and the measure $\mathrm{d}\xi_\pm$ on $\partial_\pm(X \times \Omega)$ be defined by $\mathrm{d}\xi_\pm(y, \omega) = |\omega \cdot \nu(y)| \max\{\tau_\mp(y, \omega), c\} \, \mathrm{d}\omega \, \mathrm{d}\mu(y)$. Then the trace operator*

$$\gamma_\pm \colon W^p(X \times \Omega) \to L^p\big(\partial_\pm(X \times \Omega), \mathrm{d}\xi_\pm\big), \quad v \mapsto v|_{\partial_\pm(X \times \Omega)}$$

is continuous and surjective for $p \in [1, \infty]$.

By this Lemma we see how to interpret the trace condition in the definition of the space $W_-^p(X \times \Omega)$. For functions in this space the trace is even in a smaller space, namely:

Lemma 2.3. *For $p \in [1, \infty]$ the trace operator*

$$\gamma_+ : W_-^p(X \times \Omega) \to L^p\big(\partial_+(X \times \Omega), |\omega \cdot \nu| \, d\omega \, d\mu\big), \quad v \mapsto v|_{\partial_+(X \times \Omega)}$$

is continuous.

The space $W_-^p(X \times \Omega)$ is the actual space we look for a solution of the boundary value problem (2.5)–(2.6), which we recall for convenience

$$\begin{aligned}
\omega \cdot \nabla u + \sigma_t u - S u &= q \quad \text{in } X \times \Omega \,, \\
u &= 0 \quad \text{on } \partial_-(X \times \Omega) \,.
\end{aligned} \tag{2.20}$$

For the differential operator on the left-hand side we introduce the notation L, that is,

$$\begin{aligned}
L \colon \mathcal{D}(L) \subset L^p(X \times \Omega) &\to L^p(X \times \Omega) \,, \\
u \mapsto L u &= (\omega \cdot \nabla + \sigma_t I - S) u
\end{aligned} \tag{2.21}$$

with $\mathcal{D}(L) = W_-^p(X \times \Omega)$. Using this, the boundary value problem (2.20) can be written as

$$L u = q \quad \text{with } u \in \mathcal{D}(L) \,.$$

We point out that the operator $\omega \cdot \nabla$ is unbounded from $L^p(X \times \Omega)$ into itself. In contrast, the operator $\sigma_t I$ and the scattering operator S defined in (2.4) are bounded between this space. Former statement as well as the latter for $p = \infty$ is an easy consequence of the boundedness of σ_t and σ_s and the normalization of η in (2.2). To observe the continuity of S for $p \in [1, \infty[$, we set $\widetilde{p}$ such that $1/p + 1/\widetilde{p} = 1$ and apply Hölder's inequality as well as the normalization of η:

$$\|S u\|_{L^p}^p = \int_X \int_\Omega \left| \sigma_s(x) \int_\Omega \eta(x, \omega \cdot \omega') u(x, \omega') \, d\omega' \right|^p \, d\omega \, dx$$

$$\leq \|\sigma_s\|_\infty^p \int_X \int_\Omega \left(\int_\Omega \eta(x, \omega \cdot \omega') \, d\omega' \right)^{p/\widetilde{p}} \int_\Omega \eta(x, \omega \cdot \omega') \big| u(x, \omega') \big|^p \, d\omega' \, d\omega \, dx$$

$$= \|\sigma_s\|_\infty^p \|u\|_{L^p}^p \,.$$

In the forthcoming analysis and especially in Section 6 we make use of an equivalent formulation of the boundary value problem (2.20) as an integral equation. Let us define the integral operators $\mathcal{K}, \mathcal{P} \colon L^p(X \times \Omega) \to$

$L^p(X \times \Omega)$ by

$$\mathcal{K}v(x,\omega) = \int_0^{\tau_-(x,\omega)} \exp\left(-\int_0^t \sigma_t(x - s\omega)\,\mathrm{d}s\right) Sv(x - t\omega, \omega)\,\mathrm{d}t, \quad (2.22)$$

$$\mathcal{P}v(x,\omega) = \int_0^{\tau_-(x,\omega)} \exp\left(-\int_0^t \sigma_t(x - s\omega)\,\mathrm{d}s\right) v(x - t\omega, \omega)\,\mathrm{d}t \quad (2.23)$$

for $(x,\omega) \in X \times \Omega$. Both operators are bounded. This is obvious in case $p = \infty$. If $p \in [1, \infty[$, by rewriting $\mathcal{P}$ in the form

$$\mathcal{P}v(y + r\omega, \omega) = \int_0^r \exp\left(-\int_t^r \sigma_t(y + s\omega)\,\mathrm{d}s\right) v(y + t\omega, \omega)\,\mathrm{d}t$$

with $(y,\omega) \in \partial_-(X \times \Omega)$ and $r \in [0, \tau_+(y,\omega)]$, using $\int_t^r \sigma_t(y+s\omega)\,\mathrm{d}s \geq \sigma_0 r$ and applying Lemma 2.1, we observe that

$$\|\mathcal{P}v\|_{L^p}^p = \int_\Omega \int_{\partial X_{\omega,-}} \int_0^{\tau_+(y,\omega)} \left|(\mathcal{P}v(y + r\omega, \omega))\right|^p \mathrm{d}r |\omega \cdot \nu(y)|\,\mathrm{d}\mu(y)\,\mathrm{d}\omega$$

$$\leq \frac{\mathrm{diam}(X)^{p-1}}{p\sigma_0}\left(1 - e^{-p\sigma_0 \mathrm{diam}(X)}\right) \|v\|_{L^p}^p,$$

since for almost every $(y,\omega) \in \partial_-(X \times \Omega)$ holds

$$\int_0^{\tau_+(y,\omega)} \left|(\mathcal{P}v(y + r\omega, \omega))\right|^p \mathrm{d}r$$

$$\leq \int_0^{\tau_+(y,\omega)} r^{p/\widetilde{p}} \int_0^r \exp\left(-p\int_t^r \sigma_t(y + s\omega)\,\mathrm{d}s\right) |v(y + t\omega, \omega)|^p\,\mathrm{d}t\,\mathrm{d}r$$

$$\leq \frac{\mathrm{diam}(X)^{p/\widetilde{p}}}{p\sigma_0}\left(1 - e^{-p\sigma_0 \mathrm{diam}(X)}\right) \int_0^{\tau_+(y,\omega)} |v(y + t\omega, \omega)|^p\,\mathrm{d}t.$$

Herein, $\widetilde{p}$ is again such that $1/p + 1/\widetilde{p} = 1$ and $\mathrm{diam}(X)$ denotes the diameter of the domain X. In view of $\mathcal{K} = \mathcal{P}S$, the operator $\mathcal{K}$ is also continuous.

Multiplying the radiative transfer equation at a point $(x - t\omega, \omega)$ by the integrating factor $\exp\left(-\int_0^t \sigma_t(x - s\omega)\,\mathrm{d}s\right)$ and integrating with respect to t over the interval $[0, \tau_-(x,\omega)]$ leads now to the equivalent integral equation

$$(I - \mathcal{K})u = \mathcal{P}q, \quad (2.24)$$

cf. e.g. [CS99]. Herein, we interpret $\mathcal{P}\colon L^p(X) \to L^p(X \times \Omega)$ in the canonical way via embedding of $L^p(X)$ into $L^p(X \times \Omega)$.

There is a variety of approaches to show existence and uniqueness of the solution $u \in L^p(X \times \Omega)$ of the boundary value problem (2.20) under the subcritical condition (2.18). In [**CZ67**] and [**ES13**] the integral equation (2.24) is transferred into a fixed-point problem and unique solvability is shown for this. In the former reference the cases $p = 1$ and $p = \infty$ are treated, whereas in the latter the case of general $p \in [1, \infty]$ is handled with less restrictive conditions on the coefficients than condition (2.18). Another way to show existence and uniqueness of the solution is via a reformulation of the boundary value problem as a variational problem. This approach is presented in [**Ago98**] for $p \in [1, \infty[$. A third possibility is to use the framework of semigroup theory as presented in [**DL00a, DL00b**], for instance. This seems to be the standard approach in RTE-based inverse problems, see [**Bal09, CS96**], and to be the most complete theory in L^p spaces.

The following existence and uniqueness results is recalled from §2 of Chapter XXI in [**DL00b**]:

Lemma 2.4. *For $p \in [1, \infty]$ and $q \in L^p(X \times \Omega)$ the boundary value problem (2.20) has a unique solution $u \in W_-^p(X \times \Omega)$ depending continuously on q.*

Corollary 2.5. *The operator L^{-1} from $L^p(X \times \Omega)$ into itself is bounded for $p \in [1, \infty]$. It is even bounded between $L^p(X \times \Omega)$ and $W_-^p(X \times \Omega)$.*

Finally we have all definitions and properties at hand to define the (linear and bounded) forward operator of RTE-based BLT by

$$A \colon L^p(X) \to L^p\big(\partial_+(X \times \Omega), |\omega \cdot \nu|\, \mathrm{d}\omega\, \mathrm{d}\mu\big) = \mathcal{Y}_p\,,$$
$$q \mapsto \gamma_+ L^{-1} q\,. \tag{2.25}$$

By means of this operator, the radiative transfer equation based bioluminescence tomography problem can be written as:

Problem 2.6 (RTE-based BLT Problem). *Given the measurements $g \in \mathcal{R}(A)$, find a source function $q \in L^p(X)$ such that*

$$Aq = g\,.$$

Herein, $\mathcal{R}(A)$ denotes the range of the operator A.

We finish this subsection giving two examples in which the ill-posed character of the Problem 2.6 becomes apparent. Moreover, they help to understand the RTE-based BLT better and build bridges to another well-known inverse problem, namely the single photon emission computed tomography (SPECT). These examples are standard special cases in transport theory, see for instance [**CZ67, Bal09**].

Example 2.7 (Purely absorbing media). Let X be convex with $0 \in X$ and $\sigma_s = 0$. Latter implies that $\mathcal{K} = 0$ and in this setting the RTE-based BLT problem consists of finding $q \in L^p(X)$ given

$$g(x,\omega) = \gamma_+ \mathcal{P} q(x,\omega) = \int_0^{\tau_-(x,\omega)} \exp\left(-\int_0^t \sigma_t(x - s\omega)\,\mathrm{d}s\right) q(x - t\omega)\,\mathrm{d}t$$

for $(x,\omega) \in \partial_+(X \times \Omega)$. Up to renaming of the variables, this is exactly the problem arising in SPECT, see [**NW01**]. Extending σ_t as 0 outside of X and introducing the attenuated ray transform

$$P_{\sigma_t} q(y,\omega) = \int_{\mathbb{R}} \exp\left(-\int_t^\infty \sigma_t(y + s\omega)\,\mathrm{d}s\right) q(y + t\omega)\,\mathrm{d}t$$

for $\omega \in \Omega$ and $y \in \omega^\perp = \{z \in \mathbb{R}^d \colon z \cdot \omega = 0\}$, the RTE-based BLT problem can be recasted as reconstructing q given its attenuated ray transform. For $d = 2$ inversion formulas for the attenuated ray transform were developed in [**Nat01a, Nov02**] assuming mild regularity of the coefficient σ_t and the source q.[3] By considering hyperplane by hyperplane, or slice by slice, these results can be extended to $d = 3$, see [**Nov02**]. Consequently, the operator P_{σ_t} is injective and the problem uniquely solvable.

We note that the mentioned inversion formulas can be implemented generalizing the filtered backprojection algorithm of X-ray computed tomography. For details see [**Kun01, Nat01a**].

Next we will observe that P_{σ_t} is a compact operator between suitable spaces for sufficiently smooth coefficients σ_t. So let $p = 2$. We set $T = \{(y,\omega) \in \mathbb{R}^d \times \Omega \colon y \in \omega^\perp\}$ and the space $L^2(T)$ to be the Hilbert space with norm

$$\|v\|_{L^2(T)} = \int_\Omega \int_{\omega^\perp} |v(y,\omega)|^2 \,\mathrm{d}y\,\mathrm{d}\omega.$$

Moreover, we assume that σ_t is sufficiently smooth. In [**Hei86**] it is shown that the two-dimensional attenuated Radon transform, which coincides with the attenuated ray transform P_{σ_t} in two dimensions up to notation [**NW01**], smoothes of order $\frac{1}{2}$ in Sobolev scale. The corresponding smoothing result for a broad class of weighted ray transforms, covering P_{σ_t} also in case $d = 3$, is derived in [**SU12**]. From these findings we conclude that the operator $P_{\sigma_t} \colon L^2(X) \to L^2(T)$ is compact.

---

[3]In fact, $p > 1$ and $\sigma_t \in L^\infty(\mathbb{R}^d)$ with compact support is sufficient to apply the Novikov inversion formula, cf. [**Nov02**].

In order to transfer this result back to the operator $\mathcal{P}$, we observe, similar to the proof of Lemma 2.1 above presented in [**CS99**], that

$$\int_{\omega^\perp} v\big(y + \tau_+(y,\omega)\omega\big)\,\mathrm{d}y = \int_{\partial X_{\omega,+}} v(x)|\nu(x)\cdot\omega|\,\mathrm{d}\mu(x) \qquad (2.26)$$

holds for $v \in L^1(\partial X_{\omega,+})$. Consequently,

$$\|\gamma_+ \mathcal{P}q\|_{\mathcal{Y}_2} = \|P_{\sigma_\mathrm{t}} q\|_{L^2(T)}\,.$$

With the observations above follows immediately that the forward operator A is compact and that the RTE-based BLT problem is ill-posed, at least for the special case $\sigma_\mathrm{s} = 0$ we consider in this example. However, the ill-posedness is rather mild, recalling the injectivity and the smoothing of order $\frac{1}{2}$ in Sobolev scale.

Example 2.8 (Isotropic scattering). Let X be convex and scattering be isotropic, i.e., let the scattering kernel η be independent of the angle $\omega\cdot\omega'$. In view of the directional independence of

$$Su(x) = Su(x,\omega) = \sigma_\mathrm{s}(x)\frac{1}{\mathrm{Vol}(\Omega)}\int_\Omega u(x,\omega')\,\mathrm{d}\omega'\,,$$

the radiative transfer equation becomes

$$\omega\cdot\nabla u(x,\omega) + \sigma_\mathrm{t}(x)u(x,\omega) = q(x) + Su(x) \quad \text{with } u|_{\partial_-(X\times\Omega)} = 0\,. \quad (2.27)$$

Defining the right-hand side as a function f in the spatial variable x, we have seen in the last example that f is uniquely determined by the boundary measurements of u on $\partial_+(X\times\Omega)$. Given now the function f, we obtain u solving the boundary value problem (2.27). The source term q is now easily recovered by $q = f - Su$.

Though the RTE-based BLT problem is uniquely solvable in this special case, the calculation of q uses the 'inversion' of the attenuated ray transform, a compact operator. The problem is therefore ill-posed.

The main observations of the last two examples, i.e., the unique solvability and the ill-posedness of the RTE-based problem due to the relation to the SPECT problem, can be extended to the general anisotropic case. Under a smallness assumption on the anisotropic part of the scattering kernel η in a suitable norm[4] and a smoothness assumption on σ_t, it is shown in [**BT07**] that

$$\mathcal{Q}g = (I - K)q$$

---

[4]More precisely, the Fourier coefficients of η with respect to an expansion in the angular variable have to decay sufficiently fast. See [**BT07**] for details.

holds with a contractive operator $K\colon L^2(X) \to L^2(X)$ depending linearly on η. Herein, $\mathcal{Q}\colon \mathcal{Y}_2 \to L^2(X)$ denotes the formal inverse of $\gamma_+\mathcal{P}$ obtained by an inversion formula for the attenuated ray transform, i.e., $\mathcal{Q}\gamma_+\mathcal{P} = I$. It follows that q can be reconstructed using the Neumann series

$$q = \sum_{n=0}^{\infty} K^n \mathcal{Q}g \,.$$

Moreover, in the general case where the smallness assumption does not hold, the operator K is compact. This is explained in [**BT07**] using compactness results of [**MK97**].[5] By the Fredholm alternative, cf. [**Wer07**], q is uniquely determined via

$$q = (I - K)^{-1}\mathcal{Q}g$$

if and only if 1 is not an eigenvalue of K.

2.2.2. DA-based BLT Problem. For convenience and in order to improve the numerical stability, we start by recasting the measurements in the diffusion model. By subtraction of the Robin boundary condition (2.16) from the Neumann data in (2.17), we obtain the Dirichlet boundary values

$$u_0 = 2g_0 \quad \text{on } \partial X \,. \tag{2.28}$$

Moreover, we simplify the notation by omitting the subscript 0 in u_0 and redefining $g = 2g_0$. Though the notation coincides with the one in RTE-based BLT, it will be clear from the context which model is under consideration or if we present the unified theory.

Let us now prepare the introduction of the forward operator. If not required otherwise, we will assume in the diffusion model that X is a bounded domain with sufficiently smooth boundary (at least Lipschitz continuous) and that $D, \sigma_a \in L^\infty(X)$ are bounded away from zero by constants D_0 and σ_0, respectively: $0 < D_0 \le D$ and $0 < \sigma_0 \le \sigma_a$ almost everywhere in X. When speaking of the solution u of the boundary value problem

$$-\operatorname{div}\big(D\nabla u\big) + \sigma_a u = q \quad \text{in } X \,,$$

$$u + 2D\frac{\partial u}{\partial \nu} = 0 \quad \text{on } \partial X \,, \tag{2.29}$$

---

[5]In [**BT07**] smoothness of σ_t, i.e. $\sigma_t \in C_0^2(X)$, is assumed to show compactness of K. Since for the Novikov inversion formula [**Nov02**] and the compactness results in [**MK97**] only $\sigma_t \in L^\infty(X)$, $\sigma_t > 0$ is needed, we think compactness of K holds under our general assumptions.

we refer to the weak solution. In other words, $u \in H^1(X)$ is the solution of the variational formulation

$$\int_X (D\nabla u \cdot \nabla v + \sigma_a uv)\, dx + \frac{1}{2} \int_{\partial X} uv\, d\mu = \int_X qv\, dx \quad \text{for all } v \in H^1(X).$$

In view of the Lax–Milgram lemma, see e.g. [**AH05**], the weak solution exists and is unique for every $q \in \widetilde{H}^{-1}(X)$, where $\widetilde{H}^{-1}(X)$ is the dual space of $H^1(X)$. From a standard trace theorem, cf. [**Hac92**], we know that the trace $u|_{\partial X}$ lies in $H^{1/2}(\partial X)$ and

$$\|u|_{\partial X}\|_{H^{\frac{1}{2}}(\partial X)} \leq c \|u\|_{H^1(X)}$$

holds with a constant $c \in \mathbb{R}$. As we expect noisy measurements, we weaken the regularity of the data range and define the forward operator of DA-based BLT by

$$
\begin{aligned}
A \colon L^2(X) &\to L^2(\partial X), \\
q &\mapsto u|_{\partial X},
\end{aligned}
\tag{2.30}
$$

where $u \in H^1(X)$ is the solution of the boundary value problem (2.29).

By means of this operator the diffusion approximation based bioluminescence tomography problem can be written as:

Problem 2.9 (DA-based BLT Problem). *Given the measurements $g \in \mathcal{R}(A)$, find a source function $q \in L^2(X)$ such that*

$$Aq = g.$$

We point out that Problem 2.9 is ill-posed: it suffers not only from the instability due to the compactness of A, but also from non-uniqueness. The compactness of A is obtained by the compact embedding of $H^{1/2}(\partial X)$ into $L^2(\partial X)$, see [**AH05**]. Additionally, the singular value decomposition for constant coefficients D, σ_a and a ball-shaped object X is derived in Appendix D. In Theorem D.2 it is shown that, in this special case, the singular values asymptotically decay like $n^{-3/2}$.[6]

To understand the non-uniqueness, we generalize a result on the null space of A [**WLJ04**, Proposition B.1], which we denote by $\mathcal{N}(A)$.

Lemma 2.10. *There exists an isomorphism $T \colon H^1(X) \to \widetilde{H}^{-1}(X)$ such that*

$$T\big(H_0^1(X)\big) \cap L^2(X) = \mathcal{N}(A).$$

---

[6]Since in this special case the coefficients D, σ_a as well as the boundary ∂X are smooth, the data Aq particularly lies in the smoother space $H^{3/2}(\partial X)$, cf. [**Hac92**].

If, additionally, $D \in W^{1,\infty}(X)$ holds, then

$$T\big(H_0^2(X)\big) = \mathcal{N}(A)\,.$$

PROOF. Let T be the bounded linear operator between $H^1(X)$ and its dual $\widetilde{H}^{-1}(X)$ defined by

$$u \mapsto (Tu)(v) = a(u, v)\,,$$

where a is the bilinear form corresponding to the boundary value problem (2.29), that is,

$$a(u, v) = \int_X (D\nabla u \cdot \nabla v + \sigma_\mathrm{a} uv)\,\mathrm{d}x + \frac{1}{2}\int_{\partial X} uv\,\mathrm{d}\mu\,.$$

It follows from the Lax–Milgram lemma that T is bijective.

We start showing that the specified sets are contained in the null space of A. Let q be in $T\big(H_0^1(X)\big) \cap L^2(X)$. Then we find a $u \in H_0^1(X)$ with $Tu = q$. From the definition of T follows directly that u satisfies the boundary value problem (2.29). As $u|_{\partial X} = 0$, the identity $Aq = 0$ holds.

In the case $D \in W^{1,\infty}(X)$, we see, using integration by parts, that $T\big(H_0^2(X)\big) \subset L^2(X)$. The inclusion is now an immediate consequence.

We turn to the other direction of the inclusion. Let $q \in \mathcal{N}(A)$ and u be the solution of the boundary value problem (2.29). We see directly that $q = Tu$ and $u \in H_0^1(X)$. If $D \in W^{1,\infty}(X)$, regularity theorems, see e.g. [**Hac92**], and the integration by parts formula imply $u \in H_0^2(X)$. □

So we see that the null space of A is very large. In the following example we find that even ball-shaped sources cannot be reconstructed uniquely. In addition, this example shall serve to get a better feeling of the challenges in DA-based BLT.

Example 2.11. Let $0 < \rho < R$ and X be the ball of radius R and center 0, $X = B_R(0)$, and let the source be ball-shaped with constant intensity $\lambda > 0$, $q = \lambda\chi_G$ with $G = B_\rho(0)$. We identify q with the pair (λ, ρ) in this example. Moreover, let the coefficients D, σ_a be positive constants. From regularity theorems, cf. [**Hac92**], we know that the solution u of the boundary value problem (2.29) lies in $H^2(X)$ in this case. In particular, u is continuous in $\overline{X}$ by Sobolev embedding theorems, see e.g. [**AH05**].

Now we want to express u and especially its trace in terms of the fundamental solution of the diffusion equation and then gain the crucial insight. We describe the three-dimensional case in detail and just remark the similar result in two dimensions.

In dimension $d = 3$, it is easily verified, using the representation of the Laplace operator in polar coordinates[7], that the fundamental solution of the diffusion equation with constant coefficients is given by

$$\Phi(x, y) = \frac{e^{-\widetilde{\sigma}|x-y|}}{4\pi D|x-y|} \quad \text{for } x \neq y \text{ with } \widetilde{\sigma} = \sqrt{\frac{\sigma_a}{D}}.$$

We expand the fundamental solution Φ in terms of spherical harmonics $H_{l,m}$, spherical Bessel functions j_l and spherical Hankel functions of the first kind h_l. Details on these special functions are found in the Appendices A.2 and A.3. Analogous to Theorem 2.10 in [**CK98**] we obtain:

$$\frac{e^{-\widetilde{\sigma}|x-y|}}{4\pi D|x-y|} = -\frac{\widetilde{\sigma}}{D}\sum_{l=0}^{\infty}\sum_{m=-l}^{l} h_l^{(1)}(\widetilde{\sigma}i|x|)H_{l,m}(\widehat{x})j_l(\widetilde{\sigma}i|y|)\overline{H_{l,m}(\widehat{y})} \quad (2.31)$$

for $|x| > |y|$ and with $\widehat{x} = x/|x|$ as well as $\widehat{y} = y/|y|$. This series converges absolutely and uniformly on compact subsets of $\{(x, y) \in \mathbb{R}^3 \times \mathbb{R}^3 \colon |x| > |y|\}$. Additionally, the same convergence statement is true for the series of the term by term derivatives with respect to $|x|$ and $|y|$.

In view of the smoothness of $\Phi(x, \cdot)$ in $X \setminus \{x\}$, the regularity of u and Green's second identity, we obtain similar to [**CK98**, Theorem 2.1] Green's representation formula

$$
\begin{aligned}
u(x) &= \int_X q(y)\Phi(x, y)\,\mathrm{d}y \\
&\quad + \int_{\partial X}\left[\Phi(x, y)D\frac{\partial u}{\partial \nu}(y) - u(y)D\frac{\partial}{\partial \nu(y)}\Phi(x, y)\right]\mathrm{d}\mu(y)
\end{aligned}
\quad (2.32)
$$

for $x \in \overline{X}$. We analyze the domain integral in more detail by applying the expansion of the fundamental solution (2.31) to it. Recall that $q = \lambda\chi_G$ with $G = B_\rho(0)$ and let $\rho < |x| \leq R$. Then

$$
\begin{aligned}
\int_X q(y)\Phi(x, y)\,\mathrm{d}y &= \lambda\int_{B_\rho(0)}\Phi(x, y)\,\mathrm{d}y \\
&= -\frac{\widetilde{\sigma}}{D}\lambda\int_{B_\rho(0)}\sum_{l=0}^{\infty}\sum_{m=-l}^{l} h_l^{(1)}(\widetilde{\sigma}i|x|)H_{l,m}(\widehat{x})j_l(\widetilde{\sigma}i|y|)\overline{H_{l,m}(\widehat{y})}\,\mathrm{d}y \\
&= -\frac{\widetilde{\sigma}}{D}\lambda\sum_{l=0}^{\infty}\sum_{m=-l}^{l} h_l^{(1)}(\widetilde{\sigma}i|x|)H_{l,m}(\widehat{x})\int_0^\rho r^2 j_l(\widetilde{\sigma}ir)\,\mathrm{d}r\int_{S^2}\overline{H_{l,m}(\theta)}\,\mathrm{d}\theta.
\end{aligned}
$$

---

[7]Alternatively, it can be deduced from the fundamental solution of the Helmholtz equation given e.g. in [**CK98**].

Due to the orthonormality of the spherical harmonics $H_{l,m}$, the series reduces to one summand, which we can simplify using the explicit form of the special functions of low order, cf. Appendices A.2 and A.3:

$$
\begin{aligned}
\int_X q(y)\Phi(x,y)\,\mathrm{d}y &= -\frac{\widetilde{\sigma}}{D}\lambda h_0^{(1)}(\widetilde{\sigma}i|x|)H_{0,0}(\widehat{x})\int_0^\rho r^2 j_0(\widetilde{\sigma}ir)\,\mathrm{d}r\int_{S^2}\overline{H_{0,0}(\theta)}\,\mathrm{d}\theta\\
&= -\frac{\widetilde{\sigma}}{D}\lambda h_0^{(1)}(\widetilde{\sigma}i|x|)\int_0^\rho r^2\frac{\sinh(\widetilde{\sigma}r)}{\widetilde{\sigma}r}\,\mathrm{d}r\\
&= -\frac{\lambda}{D}h_0^{(1)}(\widetilde{\sigma}i|x|)\left(\frac{\rho\cosh(\widetilde{\sigma}\rho)}{\widetilde{\sigma}}-\frac{\sinh(\widetilde{\sigma}\rho)}{\widetilde{\sigma}^2}\right)\\
&= \frac{\lambda}{\sigma_{\mathrm{a}}}\frac{\mathrm{e}^{-\widetilde{\sigma}|x|}}{\widetilde{\sigma}|x|}\big(\widetilde{\sigma}\rho\cosh(\widetilde{\sigma}\rho)-\sinh(\widetilde{\sigma}\rho)\big)
\end{aligned}
$$

for $x\in\mathbb{R}^3$ with $\rho<|x|\le R$.

Consequently, the domain integral in (2.32) takes the same value for all pairs $(\widetilde{\lambda},\widetilde{\rho})$ with

$$
\widetilde{\lambda}\big(\widetilde{\sigma}\widetilde{\rho}\cosh(\widetilde{\sigma}\widetilde{\rho})-\sinh(\widetilde{\sigma}\widetilde{\rho})\big)=\lambda\big(\widetilde{\sigma}\rho\cosh(\widetilde{\sigma}\rho)-\sinh(\widetilde{\sigma}\rho)\big)\qquad(2.33)
$$

for fixed $|x|$. We note that the function $t\mapsto t\cosh(t)-\sinh(t)$ is monotone increasing on $\mathbb{R}$. Since the boundary integrals in (2.32) are determined by the measurement and Robin boundary condition, we observe that infinite many ball-shaped sources solve the DA-based BLT problem 2.9. Given one solution (λ,ρ), a second $(\widetilde{\lambda},\widetilde{\rho})$ is obtained by increasing λ and decreasing ρ, or vice versa, such that (2.33) is satisfied.

In dimension $d=2$, an analogous result holds true. In this case the fundamental solution of the diffusion equation is given by

$$
\Phi(x,y)=\frac{1}{2\pi}K_0\big(\widetilde{\sigma}|x-y|\big)\,,
$$

where $\widetilde{\sigma}=\sqrt{\sigma_{\mathrm{a}}/D}$ as before and K_0 denotes the modified Bessel function of second kind of order 0, see Appendix A.3. Using an addition theorem for K_0, more precisely, Formula 11.41(8) in [**Wat52**], and performing the same steps as above, we obtain: The pairs (λ,ρ) and $(\widetilde{\lambda},\widetilde{\rho})$ solve the DA-based BLT problem 2.9 with identical data if

$$
\widetilde{\lambda}\widetilde{\rho}I_1(\widetilde{\sigma}\widetilde{\rho})=\lambda\rho I_1(\widetilde{\sigma}\rho)\,.
$$

Herein, I_1 is the modified Bessel function of first kind of order 1, cf. Appendix A.3.

2.3. Regularized Problem under Investigation

In the last section we have seen that the RTE-based and the DA-based BLT problem are ill-posed. Though the RTE-based BLT problem is uniquely solvable, the DA-based BLT problem suffers from non-uniqueness. Consequently, we have to incorporate both *a priori* knowledge and regularization schemes in order to get reliable reconstructions [**Kir11, Rie03**]. The approach presented here is the same as in our previously published work [**KR12**], but now covering also the RTE-based BLT problem.

We want to do this in an unified framework. The forward operator A is introduced in (2.25) and (2.30) for the transport model and diffusion model, respectively. The image space of A is denoted by $\mathcal{Y}$, that is, $\mathcal{Y} = \mathcal{Y}_1 = L^1\big(\partial_+(X \times \Omega), |\omega \cdot \nu| \, d\mu \, d\omega\big)$ in the RTE-based setting and $\mathcal{Y} = L^2(\partial X)$ if the DA-model is considered. There are two main reasons we restrict ourselves to the case $p = 1$ in RTE-based BLT. First, this is a natural choice from a physical point of view, because the L^1 norm of the solution u of the transfer equation (2.20) is the total number of photons in the object X [**Dor98**]. Second, this choice is crucial for the calculation of the domain derivative in Chapter 6, as some integrals do not exist for $p \geq 2$.

Let us begin with the discussion of the *a priori* knowledge used in the reconstruction process. As mentioned in the introduction, the bioluminescence sources are marked cells. The light intensity of every living cell is determined by the used marker, more precisely by the luciferase, and constant over the cell. Surely we are not able to resolve every cell, but still on a structure, e.g. a tumor, we may assume a constant intensity. Due to dead cells in this structure, we do not know the exact strength over it, but it will lie 'near' the intensity of the used cell line. Additionally, the source function vanishes outside of the cell structure. Consequently, we assume that the source function can be modeled by

$$q = \sum_{i=1}^{I} \lambda_i \chi_{G_i} \,, \qquad (2.34)$$

where χ_{G_i} is the characteristic function of a measurable set $G_i \subset X$ and $\lambda_i \in [\underline{\lambda}_i, \overline{\lambda}_i] = \Lambda_i$. The number I is fixed and has to be set in advance.[8]

---

[8]We note that a rough estimate of the number I of sources inside the object is obtained from the measurements. It can be approximated by the number of local maxima of the photon density on the boundary. Further discussion on this topic and a numerical example where I is overestimated are found in Section 5.2.5.

Moreover, we assume $G_i \subset X_i$ for an open subset $X_i \subset X$ since an *a priori* knowledge about the location of the sources may be available.

We use the notations $\lambda = (\lambda_1, \ldots, \lambda_I)$, $G = (G_1, \ldots, G_I)$ and $\Lambda = \Lambda_1 \times \cdots \times \Lambda_I$. In order to analyze the BLT problem and develop some reconstruction algorithms in the following, we will write it as a nonlinear operator equation $F(\lambda, G) = g$. Herein, the forward operator F is given by

$$F : \Lambda \times \mathcal{L} \quad \to \quad \mathcal{Y},$$
$$(\lambda, G) \quad \mapsto \quad \sum_{i=1}^{I} \lambda_i A \chi_{G_i} \tag{2.35}$$

with $\mathcal{L} = \mathcal{L}_{X_1} \times \cdots \times \mathcal{L}_{X_I}$ and $\mathcal{L}_{X_i}$ denoting the set of all measurable subsets of X_i.

So the inverse problem of the bioluminescence tomography in the unified notation and under these assumptions can be written as:

Problem 2.12 (Unregularized Problem). *Given the measurements g, find an intensity vector $\lambda \in \Lambda$ and a tuple of sets $G \in \mathcal{L}$ such that*

$$F(\lambda, G) = g.$$

As the nonlinear forward operator F is closely related to the linear forward operator A, the ill-posedness of Problem 2.6 and 2.9 is transferred to this problem. To face the ill-posedness, Problem 2.12 has to be regularized. For this, we combine two ideas, one from bioluminescence tomography related research and one from the field of shape optimization in inverse problems. In [**GZ10b**] a total variation (TV) regularization scheme for general sources in bioluminescence tomography is proposed. For X-ray computed tomography (CT) and SPECT a so-called Mumford–Shah like approach, which essentially penalizes the perimeter, is presented in [**RR07, KRR11**]. More precisely, we will consider regularization with the total variation, also called *BV* semi-norm (see e.g. [**ABM06**] for details), of $\sum_i \chi_{G_i}$ as penalty term, that is,

$$\sum_{i=1}^{I} |D(\chi_{G_i})|.$$

The *BV* semi-norm of $\sum_i \chi_{G_i}$ is identical with the perimeter of the sets G_i, see e.g. [**ABM06**], and will be denoted by

$$\mathrm{Per}(G) = \sum_{i=1}^{I} \mathrm{Per}(G_i) = \sum_{i=1}^{I} |D(\chi_{G_i})|. \tag{2.36}$$

We point out that in case of a Lipschitz domain G_i the perimeter coincides with the $(d-1)$-dimensional Hausdorff measure of ∂G_i.

The expected effect of the perimeter penalty term is to smooth the boundary of the reconstructed domain. In view of the identity (2.36), we observe that the regularization term coincides exactly with the one used in [**RR07, KRR11**] and that it only differs in the missing scaling with the intensities λ_i from the one of [**GZ10b**]. In using the unscaled version of the penalty term $\sum_{i=1}^{I} |\mathrm{D}(\chi_{G_i})|$ rather than $\sum_{i=1}^{I} |\mathrm{D}(\lambda_i \chi_{G_i})|$, we incorporate the nature of bioluminescence tomography: The intensity variable λ depends on the used type of marker, whereas the geometric variable G depends on the marked cells only. Hence, we treat both variables independently of each other. As we will see in Theorem 3.5 below, the use of the unscaled penalty term leads to a geometric reconstruction independent of the signal intensity, i.e., independent of the used marker, which is desired in applications. Furthermore, the penalization of the perimeter reflects the uniform growth of cell structures leading to sources with small perimeter compared to their volume.

So the problem under investigation is:

Problem 2.13 (Regularized Problem). *Minimize the Tikhonov like functional*

$$J_\alpha(\lambda, G) = \frac{1}{p}\|F(\lambda, G) - g\|_{\mathcal{Y}}^p + \alpha \mathrm{Per}(G) \qquad (2.37)$$

over $\Lambda \times \mathcal{L}$. *Herein, we set $p = 1$ in the transport and $p = 2$ in the diffusion model.*

As already mentioned above, a similar approach was used by Ramlau et al. [**RR07, KRR11**] for CT and SPECT and they called the functional of type J_α a Mumford–Shah like functional. The name refers to a similar objective functional with applications in computer vision introduced by Mumford and Shah in [**MS89**].

Let us note that in the stated framework the source q is essentially the same under changes on a set of measure zero. Also the perimeter is invariant under such alterations [**Giu84**]. Therefore, it is reasonable to consider equivalence classes of the measurable domains G_i, i.e., domains that coincide but on a set of measure zero, rather than an explicit representative.

CHAPTER 3

Analysis of the Regularized Problem

In this chapter we analyze the problem of minimizing the functional J_α defined in (2.37) in detail. The problem is non-standard, since we optimize with respect to a geometric variable, more precisely the shape, and the set of shapes is nonlinear and non-convex in general [**DZ11**]. Nevertheless, we give answers to the main questions of optimization theory. We work in the unified framework covering both models of light propagation and point out model-specific results in due course. The presentation starts with existence, stability and regularization results. Since the minimization functional J_α is neither differentiable nor one-sided directionally differentiable with respect to general measurable sets, we approximate it by smooth domains and develop an approximate variational principle based on Ekeland's ε-variational principle. We finish this chapter presenting a similar theory for star-shaped domains, where we can work on the linear space of parameterizations rather than on a set of shapes. This linear structure is essential for the numerical implementation in Chapter 5 and Chapter 7.

The theory presented in this chapter was published before in [**KR12**] in the DA-based BLT framework. These results are adapted and extended in order to fit both models. Moreover, we broaden the star-shaped framework and consider also the center points as unknowns.

3.1. Existence, Stability and Regularization Property

Let us study the minimization problem 2.13 in this section. We recall it for convenience:

$$\text{Minimize } J_\alpha(\lambda, G) = \frac{1}{p}\|F(\lambda, G) - g\|_{\mathcal{Y}}^p + \alpha \text{Per}(G) \text{ over } \Lambda \times \mathcal{L}.$$

As mentioned in the last chapter, $\mathcal{L} = \mathcal{L}_{X_1} \times \cdots \times \mathcal{L}_{X_I}$ with $\mathcal{L}_{X_i}$ denoting the set of all measurable subsets of X_i and $\Lambda = \Lambda_1 \times \cdots \times \Lambda_I$, where Λ_i are compact intervals $[\underline{\lambda}_i, \overline{\lambda}_i]$.

We proceed similar to [**RR10**], where existence, stability and regularization results for a minimization problem akin to Problem 2.13 in the L^2 setting, i.e., $\mathcal{Y}$ being an L^2 space, under an injectivity assumption was proven. However, these results are not directly applicable to either of our two models, as we consider $\mathcal{Y}$ being an L^1 space in RTE-based BLT and the DA-based BLT forward operator does not satisfy the injectivity property postulated in [**RR10**].[1] Therefore, we present a different analysis of Problem 2.13 using the constraint on $\lambda \in \Lambda$ to obtain a compactness result and covering also the L^1 case.

We point out that the following analysis is valid for every operator $F \colon \Lambda \times \mathcal{L} \to \mathcal{Z}$ that can be written in the form $B \sum \lambda_i \chi_{G_i}$, where $\mathcal{Z}$ is a Banach space and B a linear and bounded operator from $L^2(X)$ to $\mathcal{Z}$. In view of the boundedness of X, it is an easy consequence of Hölder's inequality that every linear and bounded operator from $L^1(X)$ to $\mathcal{Z}$ satisfies this continuity condition. In particular, the RTE-based BLT forward operator is also bounded from $L^2(X)$ to $\mathcal{Y}$.

3.1.1. Existence of a Solution.
When considering a minimization problem, a fundamental question is the existence of a solution. In the following theorem we observe that the Tikhonov like functional J_α possesses a minimizer:

Theorem 3.1 (Existence of a Solution). *For any $\alpha > 0$ and any $g \in \mathcal{Y}$ there exists a solution $(\lambda^*, G^*) \in \Lambda \times \mathcal{L}$ of Problem 2.13:*

$$J_\alpha(\lambda^*, G^*) \leq J_\alpha(\lambda, G) \qquad \text{for all } (\lambda, G) \in \Lambda \times \mathcal{L}.$$

---

[1]Actually, we think that the injectivity assumption in the cited article, [**RR10**, Assumption 3], can be weakened such that only injectivity needs to hold with respect to $\text{span}\{\chi_{G_i} : i = 1, \ldots, I\}$ for fixed but arbitrary $\bigcup G_i = X$. In this framework the DA-based BLT forward operator would fit if $I = 1$. But in the case $I \geq 2$ even this assumption is not satisfied. A counterexample can be constructed in a ball using a ball-shaped source enclosed by a ring-shaped source.

PROOF. The functional J_α is bounded from below by 0, so that there exists a minimizing sequence $\{(\lambda^n, G^n)\}_{n \in \mathbb{N}_0}$ decreasing in J_α and satisfying

$$\lim_{n \to \infty} J_\alpha(\lambda^n, G^n) = \inf_{(\lambda, G)} J_\alpha(\lambda, G).$$

W.l.o.g we assume that $J_\alpha(\lambda^0, G^0) < \infty$. As

$$\alpha \operatorname{Per}(G^n) \leq J_\alpha(\lambda^n, G^n) \leq J_\alpha(\lambda^0, G^0) \quad \text{for all } n \in \mathbb{N}_0,$$

and $G^n = (G_1^n, \ldots, G_I^n)$, we have

$$\operatorname{Per}(G_i^n) \leq \operatorname{Per}(G^n) \leq \frac{J_\alpha(\lambda^0, G^0)}{\alpha} \quad \text{for all } n \in \mathbb{N}_0 \text{ and } i = 1, \ldots, I.$$

Then, by the compactness of sets of finite perimeter [**DZ11**, Theorem 6.3 in Chapter 5], there exists a set $G_1^* \in \mathcal{L}_{X_1}$ such that for a subsequence $\{G_1^{n_k^1}\}_k$ holds

$$\chi_{G_1^{n_k^1}} \to \chi_{G_1^*} \quad \text{in } L^1(X) \text{ as } k \to \infty.$$

Using again the compactness of sets of finite perimeter, we find a subsequence $\{n_k^2\}_k$ of $\{n_k^1\}_k$ and a set $G_2^* \in \mathcal{L}_{X_2}$ satisfying

$$\chi_{G_2^{n_k^2}} \to \chi_{G_2^*} \quad \text{in } L^1(X) \text{ as } k \to \infty.$$

Applying this argument inductively, we obtain a subsequence $\{n_k\}_k = \{n_k^I\}_k$ such that for all i the above L^1 convergence holds, i.e.,

$$\chi_{G_i^{n_k}} \to \chi_{G_i^*} \quad \text{in } L^1(X) \text{ as } k \to \infty.$$

Since

$$0 = \lim_{k \to \infty} \|\chi_{G_i^{n_k}} - \chi_{G_i^*}\|_{L^1} = \lim_{k \to \infty} \int_X |\chi_{G_i^{n_k}} - \chi_{G_i^*}| \, \mathrm{d}x$$

$$= \lim_{k \to \infty} \int_X |\chi_{G_i^{n_k}} - \chi_{G_i^*}|^2 \, \mathrm{d}x = \lim_{k \to \infty} \|\chi_{G_i^{n_k}} - \chi_{G_i^*}\|_{L^2}^2,$$

also convergence in L^2 holds.

By the compactness of Λ, the sequence $\{\lambda^{n_k}\}_k \subset \Lambda$ possesses a convergent subsequence, also denoted by $\{\lambda^{n_k}\}_k$, with limit $\lambda^* \in \Lambda$.

Observing

$$\|\lambda_i^{n_k} \chi_{G_i^{n_k}} - \lambda_i^* \chi_{G_i^*}\|_{L^2} = \|\lambda_i^{n_k} \chi_{G_i^{n_k}} - \lambda_i^* \chi_{G_i^{n_k}} + \lambda_i^* \chi_{G_i^{n_k}} - \lambda_i^* \chi_{G_i^*}\|_{L^2}$$

$$\leq |\lambda_i^{n_k} - \lambda_i^*| \|\chi_{G_i^{n_k}}\|_{L^2} + |\lambda_i^*| \|\chi_{G_i^{n_k}} - \chi_{G_i^*}\|_{L^2},$$

we get

$$\| \sum_{i=1}^{I} \lambda_i^{n_k} \chi_{G_i^{n_k}} - \sum_{i=1}^{I} \lambda_i^* \chi_{G_i^*} \|_{L^2} \leq \sum_{i=1}^{I} \| \lambda_i^{n_k} \chi_{G_i^{n_k}} - \lambda_i^* \chi_{G_i^*} \|_{L^2} \to 0 \text{ as } k \to \infty .$$

The first term in J_α is lower semicontinuous, since A is a bounded linear operator and the norm is lower semicontinuous. Moreover, the perimeter is lower semicontinuous, cf. [**ABM06**, Proposition 10.1.1]. Combining these results, leads to

$$J_\alpha(\lambda^*, G^*) \leq \liminf_{k \to \infty} J_\alpha(\lambda^{n_k}, G^{n_k}) ,$$

which implies

$$J_\alpha(\lambda^*, G^*) = \inf_{(\lambda, G)} J_\alpha(\lambda, G) .$$

Thus, (λ^*, G^*) is a solution of the minimization problem 2.13. □

3.1.2. Stability. The regularization term is introduced into the functional J_α to face the ill-posedness of the BLT problem. We see in the sequel that this indeed stabilizes the reconstruction in our geometric approach. The argument is based on the following lemma taken from [**RR10**] and naturally generalized to the space $\mathcal{Y}$ rather than an L^2 space.

Lemma 3.2. *Let $g_n \to g$ in $\mathcal{Y}$ as $n \to \infty$ and denote by J_α^n the functional J_α with g replaced by g_n. Further, let (λ^n, G^n) be a minimizer of J_α^n over $\Lambda \times \mathcal{L}$. Then there exists a constant $C > 0$ with*

$$\mathrm{Per}(G^n) \leq C \quad \text{for all } n .$$

Theorem 3.3 (Stability). *Let $g_n \to g$ in $\mathcal{Y}$ as $n \to \infty$ and let (λ^n, G^n) minimize*

$$J_\alpha^n(\lambda, G) = \frac{1}{p} \| F(\lambda, G) - g_n \|_{\mathcal{Y}}^p + \alpha \mathrm{Per}(G) \quad \text{over } \Lambda \times \mathcal{L} .$$

Then there exists a subsequence $\{(\lambda^{n_k}, G^{n_k})\}_k$ converging to a minimizer $(\lambda^*, G^*) \in \Lambda \times \mathcal{L}$ of J_α in the sense that

$$\sum_{i=1}^{I} \| \lambda_i^{n_k} \chi_{G_i^{n_k}} - \lambda_i^* \chi_{G_i^*} \|_{L^2} \to 0 \quad \text{as } k \to \infty . \tag{3.1}$$

Furthermore, every convergent subsequence of $\{(\lambda^n, G^n)\}_n$ converges as defined by (3.1) to a minimizer of J_α.

PROOF. From Lemma 3.2 we derive the uniform boundedness of the perimeter of G^n. As in the proof of Theorem 3.1 we find a subsequence

$\{(\lambda^{n_k}, G^{n_k})\}_k$ and a pair (λ^*, G^*) such that $\chi_{G_i^{n_k}}$ converges to $\chi_{G_i^*}$ in L^1 as well as $\lambda_i^{n_k} \chi_{G_i^{n_k}}$ to $\lambda_i^* \chi_{G_i^*}$ in L^2 for every i.

It remains to show that the limit is indeed a minimizer of J_α. Since the operator A is bounded, we have

$$\|\sum_{i=1}^{I} \lambda_i^{n_k} A\chi_{G_i^{n_k}} - g_{n_k}\|_{\mathcal{Y}} - \|\sum_{i=1}^{I} \lambda_i^* A\chi_{G_i^*} - g\|_{\mathcal{Y}}$$

$$\leq \sum_{i=1}^{I} \|\lambda_i^{n_k} A\chi_{G_i^{n_k}} - \lambda_i^* A\chi_{G_i^*}\|_{\mathcal{Y}} + \|g - g_{n_k}\|_{\mathcal{Y}} \to 0$$

as $k \to \infty$. Using this convergence, the lower semicontinuity of the perimeter and the minimal property of (λ^{n_k}, G^{n_k}), we conclude that

$$J_\alpha(\lambda^*, G^*) \leq \liminf_{k \to \infty} J_\alpha^{n_k}(\lambda^{n_k}, G^{n_k}) \leq \lim_{k \to \infty} J_\alpha^{n_k}(\lambda, G) = J_\alpha(\lambda, G)$$

for any $(\lambda, G) \in \Lambda \times \mathcal{L}$. Thus, the limit (λ^*, G^*) is a minimizer of J_α. $\square$

Remark 3.4. In the transport model we might be interested in a convergence result like (3.1) in $L^1(X)$ instead of $L^2(X)$. This follows immediately from Hölder's inequality and the boundedness of X.

3.1.3. Regularization Property. Combining the above ideas of constructing a convergent subsequence with the regularization result from [**RR10**] in a straightforward manner, we get that the proposed geometric approach is indeed a regularization method.

Theorem 3.5 (Regularization Property). *Let g be in the range of F and choose the regularization parameter according to $\delta \mapsto \alpha(\delta)$ with*

$$\alpha(\delta) \to 0 \quad and \quad \frac{\delta^p}{\alpha(\delta)} \to 0 \quad as \ \delta \to 0\,,$$

where p is the exponent of the residual term in J_α. In addition, let $\{\delta_n\}_n$ be a positive null sequence and $\{g_n\}_n$ such that

$$\|g_n - g\|_{\mathcal{Y}} \leq \delta_n\,.$$

Then, with the notation of Theorem 3.3, the sequence $\{(\lambda^n, G^n)\}$ of minimizers of $J_{\alpha(\delta_n)}^n$ possesses a subsequence converging to a solution (λ^+, G^+) of the unregularized problem 2.12 with G^+ having minimal perimeter:

$$G^+ = \arg\min\{\mathrm{Per}(G)\colon G \in \mathcal{L} \ s.t. \ \exists \lambda \in \Lambda \ with \ F(\lambda, G) = g\}\,. \quad (3.2)$$

Furthermore, every convergent subsequence of $\{(\lambda^n, G^n)\}_n$ converges in terms of (3.1) to a solution $(\lambda^\dagger, G^\dagger)$ of Problem 2.12 with property (3.2).

3.2. Approximation by Smooth Domains

From the last section we know that there exists a minimizer of the functional J_α defined in (2.37). However, we have so far no characterization of the minimizer at hand which we can use as basis for an optimization method. Connected to that is the question how to modify a given shape G in order to decrease the functional value $J_\alpha(\lambda, G)$. We tackle these issues by approximating measurable sets by sets with smooth boundary and differentiate the forward operator with respect to smooth shapes. From latter calculations we also obtain the derivative of J_α with respect to smooth shapes, even though it is only a one-sided directional derivative in the transport model due to the non-differentiability of the L^1 norm.

In this section we only present the general framework, covering both models. In Chapter 4 and Chapter 6, where we handle the diffusion and transport model exclusively, we go into more detail.

So let us assume in this section[2] that

$$G_i \in \mathcal{G}_i = \left\{ \Gamma \subset X_i \colon \partial\Gamma \in C^2 \right\}.$$

We introduce the shorthand notation of the last relation

$$G \in \mathcal{G} = \mathcal{G}_1 \times \cdots \times \mathcal{G}_I.$$

In view of the following lemma, cf. [**Giu84**, Theorem 1.24], the smoothness assumption on G appears not to be too restrictive.

Lemma 3.6. *Let Γ be a bounded measurable set in $\mathbb{R}^d$ with finite perimeter. Then there exists a sequence $\{\Gamma^n\}_n$ of sets with C^∞ boundaries such that*

$$\int_{\mathbb{R}^d} |\chi_{\Gamma^n} - \chi_\Gamma| \, \mathrm{d}x \to 0 \quad \text{and} \quad \mathrm{Per}(\Gamma^n) \to \mathrm{Per}(\Gamma) \quad \text{as } n \to \infty.$$

3.2.1. The Domain Derivative. The derivative with respect to a smooth shape we use in this thesis is a natural extension of the Fréchet derivative in Banach spaces. We call it *domain derivative* going back to [**Kir93**, **HR96**]. In the literature it is also known just as Fréchet derivative [**DZ11**, **Hyv07**].

Following [**Het99**, **Sim80**], we consider variations Γ_h of the set $\Gamma \in \mathcal{S} = \{\Sigma \subset X \colon \partial\Sigma \in C^2\}$ caused by a vector field $h \in C_0^1(X, \mathbb{R}^d)$:

$$\Gamma_h = \{x + h(x) \colon x \in \Gamma\}.$$

---

[2]The assumption may be weakened, but we impose the stronger one to avoid technical difficulties.

If h is small enough, say if $\|h\|_{C^1} < 1/2$, then the vector field h is a contraction and thus

$$\varphi = \mathrm{id} + h$$

a diffeomorphism on X, where id is the identity map. In this case, $\Gamma_h \subset X$. Moreover, $\Gamma_h \in \mathcal{S}$ if $h \in C_0^2(X, \mathbb{R}^d)$.

The domain derivative of a mapping $\Phi\colon \mathcal{S} \to \mathcal{Z}$ about a point Γ, where $\mathcal{Z}$ is a Banach space, is the linear operator $\Phi'(\Gamma) \in \mathcal{L}(C_0^1, \mathcal{Z})$ satisfying

$$\|\Phi(\Gamma_h) - \Phi(\Gamma) - \Phi'(\Gamma)h\|_{\mathcal{Z}} = \mathrm{o}(\|h\|_{C^1}).$$

We point out the obvious analogy to the well known Fréchet derivative in Banach spaces. The only difference is that the maps, Φ etc., are evaluated at a set, but all the variations are performed in the Banach space $C_0^1(X, \mathbb{R}^d)$.

We note that there are also other ways to define a derivative with respect to the shape. The most prominent are the shape derivative based on the velocity method [**SZ92, DZ11**] and the topological derivative [**CR08, LHFS13**]. The former uses transformations along velocity flows, rather than perturbations of the identity as above. However, the first-order domain derivative and first-order shape derivative based on the velocity method coincide if the domain derivative exists [**DZ11**]. The topological derivative quantifies the sensitivity of the objective functional to a small change in the topology of the searched-for shape, e.g. by the creation of a small source of predefined form. We point out that the topological derivative is only defined for functionals, at least to our knowledge. In contrast to the domain derivative, no *a priori* assumption on the topology of the searched-for shape is needed. Though there exist iterative schemes based entirely on the topological derivative [**CR12**], the topological derivative is often only used to find an initial guess for a shape optimization method based on the domain or shape derivative mentioned above, see [**HLN12, CD12**] for examples. Moreover, for certain functionals, for instance for integrals of shape dependent solutions of elliptic boundary value problems, the topological derivative can be calculated given the domain or shape derivative [**NFTP03**].

The domain derivatives of the model dependent forward operators are derived in the model-specific parts, more precisely in Chapter 4 for the DA setting and in Chapter 6 in the RTE framework. As the penalty term is the same in both models, we finish this subsection calculating the domain derivative of it, i.e., of the perimeter operator $\mathrm{Per}\colon \mathcal{S} \to \mathbb{R}$ given by

$$\mathrm{Per}(\Gamma) = |\mathrm{D}(\chi_\Gamma)|. \tag{3.3}$$

Since the boundary of Γ is in particular Lipschitz, we obtain by Remark 10.3.3 of [**ABM06**]

$$\mathrm{Per}(\Gamma) = \mathcal{H}^{d-1}(\partial\Gamma) = \int_{\partial\Gamma} 1\,\mathrm{d}\mu\,, \qquad (3.4)$$

where $\mathcal{H}^{d-1}$ denotes the $(d-1)$-dimensional Hausdorff measure. Using the right identity of (3.4) and the explanations in [**Sim80**], we find:

Lemma 3.7 (Domain Derivative of Per). *The domain derivative of the perimeter defined in* (3.3) *in direction* $h \in C_0^1(X,\mathbb{R}^d)$ *about* $\Gamma \in \mathcal{S}$ *is given by*

$$\partial_\Gamma \mathrm{Per}(\Gamma)h = \int_{\partial\Gamma} \mathrm{H}_{\partial\Gamma} h_\nu \,\mathrm{d}\mu\,. \qquad (3.5)$$

Herein, $\mathrm{H}_{\partial\Gamma}$ *denotes the additive curvature of* $\partial\Gamma$, *which is* $d-1$ *times the mean curvature of* $\partial\Gamma$.

PROOF. See [**Sim80**, Theorem 5.1] for the case $h \in C_0^2(X,\mathbb{R}^d)$. This result is extendable to $h \in C_0^1(X,\mathbb{R}^d)$ by arguments found in [**DZ11**, Chapter 9]. $\qquad\square$

3.2.2. Approximate Variational Principle.

Knowing the sense of the derivative with respect to a shape, at least on a dense subsets of shapes, we elaborate now an approximate variational principle based on Ekeland's ε-variational principle. This result provides the basis for estimates on the derivative and one-sided directional derivative of J_α at smooth shapes near the optimal shape in the diffusion and the transport model, respectively. These consequences are presented in the model specific parts, more precisely in Chapter 4 and Chapter 6, respectively.

Though we derive the domain derivative of the forward operators below, which implies the continuity with respect to a perturbation h, we present a direct verification at this point already. To this end, we state an estimate on the volume of the symmetric difference of a domain and its perturbed version. This lemma will also be useful in the further analysis in Chapter 4 and Chapter 6.

Lemma 3.8. *Let* $\Gamma \in \mathcal{S}$ *be a set with finite perimeter and* $h \in C_0^1(X,\mathbb{R}^d)$ *a vector field with* $\|h\|_{C^1}$ *sufficiently small. As usual, let* Γ_h *denote the perturbed set. Then the following estimates hold for the volume of the symmetric difference* $\Gamma \Delta \Gamma_h = (\Gamma\backslash\Gamma_h) \cup (\Gamma_h\backslash\Gamma)$:

    (a) If $d = 2$, *then*

$$\mathrm{Vol}(\Gamma\Delta\Gamma_h) \le 2\mathrm{Per}(\Gamma)\|h\|_\infty\,.$$

(b) In case $d = 3$ we additionally assume that Γ is the union of N disjoint connected sets. Then

$$\mathrm{Vol}(\Gamma \Delta \Gamma_h) \leq 2\mathrm{Per}(\Gamma)\|h\|_\infty + \frac{8\pi N}{3}\|h\|_\infty^3 \,.$$

PROOF. Let Γ be the (countable) union of the disjoint connected sets Γ^n. For each n we consider the tube T_h^n with radius $\|h\|_\infty$ around the boundary $\partial \Gamma^n$. Obviously, $\Gamma \Delta \Gamma_h \subset \bigcup_n T_h^n$ and thus

$$\mathrm{Vol}(\Gamma \Delta \Gamma_h) \leq \sum_n \mathrm{Vol}(T_h^n) \,.$$

In [**Wey39**] an upper bound for the volumes of tubes of type T_h^n is given:

$$\mathrm{Vol}(T_h^n) \leq \begin{cases} 2\mathrm{Per}(\Gamma^n)\|h\|_\infty \,, & d = 2 \,, \\ 2\mathrm{Per}(\Gamma^n)\|h\|_\infty + \widetilde{C}_{\Gamma^n}\|h\|_\infty^3 \,, & d = 3 \,. \end{cases}$$

This inequality is sharp if no cross-sections overlap. The constant $\widetilde{C}_{\Gamma^n}$ is an invariant of Γ^n and is calculated in [**BG88**, Corollary 7.5.5] to be

$$\widetilde{C}_{\Gamma^n} = \frac{8\pi}{3}(1 - \gamma^n) \,,$$

where γ^n denotes the genus of Γ^n. It can be bounded by

$$\widetilde{C}_{\Gamma^n} \leq \frac{8\pi}{3} =: C \,.$$

As the Γ^n's are disjoint, $\mathrm{Per}(\Gamma) = \sum_n \mathrm{Per}(\Gamma^n)$. If $d = 2$, we finally observe that

$$\mathrm{Vol}(\Gamma \Delta \Gamma_h) \leq \sum_n \mathrm{Vol}(T_h^n) \leq \sum_n 2\mathrm{Per}(\Gamma^n)\|h\|_\infty = 2\mathrm{Per}(\Gamma)\|h\|_\infty \,.$$

For $d = 3$ we end with

$$
\begin{aligned}
\mathrm{Vol}(\Gamma \Delta \Gamma_h) &\leq \sum_{n=1}^N \mathrm{Vol}(T_h^n) \\
&\leq \sum_{n=1}^N \big(2\mathrm{Per}(\Gamma^n)\|h\|_\infty + C\|h\|_\infty^3\big) \\
&\leq 2\mathrm{Per}(\Gamma)\|h\|_\infty + CN\|h\|_\infty^3 \,.
\end{aligned}
\tag{3.6}
$$

$\square$

In view of

$$\|\chi_{\Gamma_h} - \chi_\Gamma\|_{L^1} = \|\chi_{\Gamma_h} - \chi_\Gamma\|_{L^2}^2 = \mathrm{Vol}(\Gamma \Delta \Gamma_h)$$

together with the previous lemma, the continuity of the forward operator as
well as the domain differentiability of the perimeter term, we observe that
the map $h \mapsto J_\alpha(\lambda, G_h)$ is continuous from C^1 to $\mathbb{R}$ under the assumptions
that $G \in \mathcal{G}$ has finite perimeter and that in case $d = 3$ each component of G
is the disjoint union of at most a finite number of connected domains. This
technical assumption is needed in (3.6), but quite naturally interpreted: in
each predefined X_i there are at most finitely many different sources with
connected support. Later, after the calculation of the domain derivative,
the continuity of J_α follows from the domain differentiability. In this case,
the additional assumption in three dimensions can be dropped to obtain
continuity.

Our following approximate variational principle is formulated for a
general subspace $\mathcal{V}$ of C^2. We use the space C^2, instead of C^1, to ensure
that the perturbed domain has C^2 boundary. In this case, the domain
derivative about the perturbed domain is well-defined. The subspace $\mathcal{V}$
is introduced to obtain the statement also in a smaller Hilbert space, in
which we apply an optimization scheme later. The proof of the principle
is basically an application and modification of the findings from [**Eke74,
Eke79**].

Let us introduce the following notation: For $h \in C_0^2(X, \mathbb{R}^d)^I$ and
$G \in \mathcal{G}$ we define

$$G_h := (\mathrm{id} + h)(G) = \left((\mathrm{id} + h_1)(G_1), \ldots, (\mathrm{id} + h_I)(G_I)\right).$$

Moreover, we use the norm

$$\|(k, h)\|_{\mathbb{R}^I \times \mathcal{V}} = \sqrt{\|k\|_2^2 + \|h\|_{\mathcal{V}}^2}$$

for elements (k, h) of $\mathbb{R}^I \times \mathcal{V}$.

Theorem 3.9 (Approximate Variational Principle). *Let (λ^*, G^*) be a
minimizer of J_α. Further, let $\varepsilon > 0$ and $G^\varepsilon \in \mathcal{G}$ be such that*

$$J_\alpha(\lambda^*, G^\varepsilon) \leq J_\alpha(\lambda^*, G^*) + \varepsilon. \tag{3.7}$$

*In case $d = 3$, assume that each component of G^ε is a finite union of
disjoint connected domains. Additionally, let $\mathcal{V}$ be a Banach space with
$\mathcal{V} \subset \prod_{i=1}^I C_0^2(X_i, \mathbb{R}^d)$ and $\|v\|_{C^2} \leq C\|v\|_{\mathcal{V}}$ for a constant $C > 0$.*

*Then for every $\gamma \in \,]0, \frac{1}{2C}[$ there exist a vector field $v \in \mathcal{V}$ and an
intensity $\lambda^\varepsilon \in \Lambda$ with*

$$\|(\lambda^\varepsilon - \lambda^*, v)\|_{\mathbb{R}^I \times \mathcal{V}} \leq \gamma \tag{3.8}$$

such that the perturbed domain $G_v^\varepsilon = (\mathrm{id} + v)(G^\varepsilon)$ *and the intensity* λ^ε
satisfy

$$J_\alpha(\lambda^\varepsilon, G_v^\varepsilon) \leq J_\alpha(\lambda^*, G^\varepsilon),\tag{3.9}$$

$$J_\alpha(\lambda^\varepsilon, G_v^\varepsilon) - \frac{\varepsilon}{\gamma}\|(k,h)\|_{\mathbb{R}^I \times \mathcal{V}} < J_\alpha(\lambda^\varepsilon + k, G_{v+h}^\varepsilon)\tag{3.10}$$

for all $\lambda^\varepsilon + k \in \Lambda \setminus \{\lambda^\varepsilon\}$ *and* $v + h \in \mathcal{V} \setminus \{v\}$ *with* $\|v + h\|_{\mathcal{V}} \leq \frac{1}{2C}$.

PROOF. Let us consider the ball $B_{\frac{1}{2C}} = \{w \in \mathcal{V}: \|w\|_{\mathcal{V}} \leq \frac{1}{2C}\}$ and the functional $\Psi\colon \Lambda \times B_{\frac{1}{2C}} \to \mathbb{R}$ mapping (λ, w) to $J_\alpha(\lambda, G_w^\varepsilon)$. Then Ψ is continuous, since

$$\Psi(\lambda + k, w + h) - \Psi(\lambda, w)$$
$$= J_\alpha(\lambda + k, G_{w+h}^\varepsilon) - J_\alpha(\lambda, G_{w+h}^\varepsilon) + J_\alpha(\lambda, G_{w+h}^\varepsilon) - J_\alpha(\lambda, G_w^\varepsilon)$$
$$= J_\alpha(\lambda + k, G_{w+h}^\varepsilon) - J_\alpha(\lambda, G_{w+h}^\varepsilon) + J_\alpha\big(\lambda, (G_w^\varepsilon)_{\widetilde{h}}\big) - J_\alpha(\lambda, G_w^\varepsilon)$$

for all $\lambda, \lambda + k \in \Lambda$ and $w, w + h \in B_{\frac{1}{2C}}$ with $\widetilde{h} = h \circ (\mathrm{id} + w)^{-1}$, and since J_α is continuous in both variables, as shown above. The existence of a $(\lambda^\varepsilon, v) \in \Lambda \times \mathcal{V}$ satisfying the first three estimates (3.8), (3.9) and (3.10) is a direct consequence of Ekeland's ε-variational principle [**Eke74**, Theorem 1.1]. □

Remark 3.10. We point out that for all $\varepsilon > 0$ we always find a $G^\varepsilon \in \mathcal{G}$ satisfying (3.7). This follows directly from the density result in Lemma 3.6 and the continuity of the norm term in J_α. Moreover, the additional condition on G^ε for $d = 3$ is satisfied if each component of the minimizer G^* is a finite union of disjoint connected sets.

In Chapter 4 and Chapter 6 we give corollaries to Theorem 3.9 that estimate the derivative of J_α. The estimates are approximations to well-known necessary conditions on minimizers. For the diffusion model we see in Chapter 4 that the domain derivative of J_α exists and its operator norm becomes arbitrary small near the minimizer of J_α. In the RTE-based BLT framework all one-sided directional derivatives of J_α are bounded below by $-\varepsilon$ for arbitrary small $\varepsilon > 0$. Details are stated in Chapter 6.

3.3. Theory for Star-shaped Domains

In this section we set the stage for the use of optimization methods to solve the minimization problem 2.13. All usual optimization methods require an underlying linear space, but the set of shapes is nonlinear. A standard and intuitive way to overcome this issue is working with pa-rameterizations of the boundary [**CDKT13, HT11, Het99**]. Here we

choose the framework of boundary parameterizations of star-shaped domains, as it is sufficiently general, analytically well-established and rather
implementation-friendly, see Chapter 5 and Chapter 7. Below we elaborate a self-contained theory for star-shaped domains: we show, for instance, that the minimizing domain is star-shaped and that the approximate variational principle yields almost critical smooth domains which
are star-shaped as well. These results do not immediately follow from our
general findings of the previous sections.

An alternative to our approach is the parameterization of the boundary
via closed curves as in [**HT11**], but then more effort is needed to prevent
self-intersections of the boundary. An entire different way to obtain a
linear structure on the set of shapes is to use level set techniques, see
e.g. [**BO05, DCL12, Set99**]. In this method, the shapes are represented
by the level set of a continuous function and the analysis and calculation
is performed on this level set function. It has the advantage over the
parameterization of the boundary that topological changes are possible
in general. However, we concentrate on the boundary parameterization
of star-shaped domains for above stated reasons. Our results might be
extended to other boundary parameterizations or to the level set approach,
but that is beyond the scope of this work.

Having mentioned the level set technique, we point out that the domain derivative can be used to obtain the velocity for the evolution of the
level set function [**BO05**] and that the domain derivative is closely related
to the level set derivative[3] [**LS03**].

We begin introducing the assumptions and the notation in the star-
shaped framework. Let the X_i's be closed and convex. Further, we consider only domains G_i that are star-shaped with respect to a point $m_i \in X_i$.
In other words, we suppose that for every point $m_i \in X_i$ there exists a
function $r_{X_i,m_i} \in L^\infty(S^{d-1})$ such that $r_{X_i,m_i}(\theta)\theta + m_i, \theta \in S^{d-1}$, is a parameterization of the boundary ∂X_i. Furthermore, we restrict our search
for the support of the ith source to the set

$$\mathcal{L}_i^\star = \{\Gamma \subset X_i \colon \Gamma \text{ is a star-shaped domain with respect to a point } m_i\},$$

which can be identified with

$$\mathcal{R}_i = \{(r_i, m_i) \in L^\infty(S^{d-1}) \times X_i \colon 0 \le r \le r_{X_i,m_i} \text{ a.e.}\}.$$

---

[3]The level set derivative is the generalized derivative with respect to the level set
function, cf. [**LS03**].

We will use the abbreviations

$$\mathcal{L}^{\star} = \prod_{i=1}^{I} \mathcal{L}_i^{\star} \quad \text{and} \quad \mathcal{R} = \prod_{i=1}^{I} \mathcal{R}_i$$

and additionally

$$(r, m) \in \mathcal{R} \quad \text{iff} \quad (r_i, m_i) \in \mathcal{R}_i \, .$$

For $(r, m) \in \mathcal{R}$ we understand $J_\alpha(\lambda, r, m)$ to be the value of J_α evaluated at $(\lambda, G_{(r,m)})$, where $G_{(r,m)} \in \mathcal{L}^{\star}$ is the tuple of domains represented by (r, m). In the same way we understand expressions like $F(\lambda, r, m)$ and $\mathrm{Per}(r, m) = \mathrm{Per}(r)$.

With these definitions at hand, we are able to state the minimization problem under consideration:

$$\text{Minimize} \quad J_\alpha(\lambda, r, m) \quad \text{over} \quad \Lambda \times \mathcal{R} \, . \tag{3.11}$$

Now, as we have an underlying linear structure, we can address the question of convexity of the functional J_α. Convexity of the minimization functional is an important property, since then every stationary point is a global minimizer. We will answer this question giving a counterexample for DA-based BLT:

Example 3.11 (Non-convexity). Let $d = 3$ and $D = \sigma_{\mathrm{a}} = 1$ be constant. Moreover, let X be the ball centered at the origin with radius $R > 0$ and $I = 1$. We consider ball-shaped sources centered at the origin with constant intensity $\lambda > 0$, $q = \lambda \chi_G$ with $G = B_\rho(0)$ and $0 < \rho < R$. So we are in a special case of Example 2.11. To show the non-convexity of J_α, we calculate $J_\alpha(\lambda, \rho, 0) = J_\alpha\big(\lambda, B_\rho(0)\big)$ explicitly and then show that the Hessian of J_α is indefinite.

In a first step we derive an explicit representation of the solution u of the diffusion equation (2.29) via the Green's function. Let Φ be the fundamental solution, which has the form

$$\Phi(x, y) = -\sum_{l=0}^{\infty} \sum_{k=-l}^{l} h_l^{(1)}(i|x|) H_{l,k}(\hat{x}) j_l(i|y|) \overline{H_{l,k}(\hat{y})} \tag{3.12}$$

for $|y| < |x| \le R$, where $\hat{z} = z/|z|$, compare equation (2.31). It is well known [**RR04**] that the function $G(x, y) = \Phi(x, y) + \phi(x, y)$ is the Green's function of the considered boundary value problem if for all $y \in X$

$$-\Delta\phi(\,\cdot\,, y) + \phi(\,\cdot\,, y) = 0 \quad \text{in } X \, ,$$

$$\phi(\,\cdot\,, y) + 2\frac{\partial}{\partial \nu}\phi(\,\cdot\,, y) = -\Phi(\,\cdot\,, y) - 2\frac{\partial}{\partial \nu}\Phi(\,\cdot\,, y) \quad \text{on } \partial X \, . \tag{3.13}$$

Using the representation of the Laplace operator in polar coordinates[4], it is easily verified that $j_l(i|x|)H_{l,k}(\hat{x})$ is a smooth solution of the homogeneous diffusion equation with coefficients $D = \sigma_a = 1$. Therefore, we make the ansatz

$$\phi(x, y) = \sum_{l=0}^{\infty} \sum_{k=-l}^{l} \phi_{l,k}(y) j_l(i|x|) H_{l,k}(\hat{x}). \qquad (3.14)$$

The coefficients $\phi_{l,k}$ have to be chosen in such a way that $\phi(\cdot, y)$ satisfies the boundary condition in (3.13). The normal derivative of the fundamental solution for $x \in \partial X = \partial B_R(0)$ is obtained by differentiating (3.12):

$$\frac{\partial}{\partial\nu(x)}\Phi(x, y) = -i\sum_{l=0}^{\infty}\sum_{k=-l}^{l} h_l^{(1)\prime}(i|x|)H_{l,k}(\hat{x})j_l(i|y|)\overline{H_{l,k}(\hat{y})}.$$

Consequently, we set

$$\phi_{l,k}(y) = \frac{2ih_l^{(1)\prime}(iR) + h_l^{(1)}(iR)}{2ij_l'(iR) + j_l(iR)}j_l(i|y|)\overline{H_{l,k}(\hat{y})}$$

for $y \in X$ and observe that the boundary condition in (3.13) is fulfilled term by term. We note that $\phi_{l,k}$ is well-defined, since all zeros of the spherical Bessel functions are real [**Leb73**, Theorem 5.13.4]. Applying similar techniques as in the proof of Theorem 2.10 in [**CK98**], we see that the series in (3.14) converges absolutely and uniformly on any compact subset of $\overline{X} \times X$. Moreover, the same convergence statement is true for the series of the term by term derivatives with respect to $|x|$ and $|y|$. It follows that $G(x, y) = \Phi(x, y) + \phi(x, y)$ is a Green's function.

The Green's representation formula (2.32) for the solution u of (2.29) now becomes, by adding Green's second identity applied to ϕ and u:

$$u(x) = \int_X q(y)G(x, y)\,dy = \int_X q(y)\big(\Phi(x, y) + \phi(x, y)\big)\,dy. \qquad (3.15)$$

Inserting the series expansions (3.12) and (3.14) for Φ and ϕ, respectively, we can simplify the domain integral as in Example 2.11. We obtain

$$u(x) = \lambda(\rho\cosh\rho - \sinh\rho)\left(e^{-R} + c_0\sinh R\right)\frac{1}{R} \qquad (3.16)$$

---

[4]Like in Example 2.11, it can alternatively be deduced from a similar statement for the Helmholtz equation in [**CK98**].

for $x \in \partial X = \partial B_R(0)$, where

$$c_0 = \frac{2ih_0^{(1)\prime}(iR) + h_0^{(1)}(iR)}{2ij_0'(iR) + j_0(iR)} = \frac{e^{-R}(R+2)}{2R\cosh R + (R-2)\sinh R}\,.$$

In the next step we use the explicit representation (3.16) of u to show that $J_\alpha(\lambda, \rho)$ is not convex, by observing that the Hessian of J_α is indefinite. We introduce the abbreviations

$$c_R = \left(e^{-R} + c_0\sinh R\right)\frac{1}{R} \quad \text{and} \quad \psi(\rho) = \rho\cosh\rho - \sinh\rho$$

as well as

$$a = 2\pi R^2 c_R^2\,, \quad b = -R^2 c_R \int_{S^2} g(R\theta)\,\mathrm{d}\theta\,, \quad c = \frac{1}{2}R^2 \int_{S^2} g(R\theta)^2\,\mathrm{d}\theta\,.$$

As u is positive on the boundary, also the measurement g has to be positive. In view of $c_R > 0$, we have $b < 0$. Now, the functional J_α can be expressed as

$$J_\alpha(\lambda, \rho) = \frac{1}{2}\|c_R\lambda\psi(\rho) - g\|_{L^2}^2 + \alpha\mathrm{Per}(\rho)$$
$$= a\lambda^2\psi(\rho)^2 + b\lambda\psi(\rho) + c + \alpha 4\pi\rho^2\,.$$

We calculate the gradient and the Hessian of J_α:

$$\nabla J_\alpha(\lambda, \rho) = 2a\begin{pmatrix} \lambda\psi(\rho)^2 \\ \lambda^2\psi'(\rho)\psi(\rho) \end{pmatrix} + b\begin{pmatrix} \psi(\rho) \\ \lambda\psi'(\rho) \end{pmatrix} + \alpha\begin{pmatrix} 0 \\ 8\pi\rho \end{pmatrix}$$

and

$$\mathcal{H}J_\alpha(\lambda, \rho) = 2a\begin{pmatrix} \psi(\rho)^2 & 2\lambda\psi'(\rho)\psi(\rho) \\ 2\lambda\psi'(\rho)\psi(\rho) & \lambda^2\left(\psi'(\rho)^2 + \psi''(\rho)\psi(\rho)\right) \end{pmatrix}$$
$$+ b\begin{pmatrix} 0 & \psi'(\rho) \\ \psi'(\rho) & \lambda\psi''(\rho) \end{pmatrix} + \alpha\begin{pmatrix} 0 & 0 \\ 0 & 8\pi \end{pmatrix}$$
$$= 2aA_1 + bA_2 + \alpha A_3\,.$$

It is well-known that a real symmetric 2×2 matrix is indefinite if and only if its determinant is negative. After some algebraic manipulations, the determinant of $2aA_1 + bA_2$ reads

$$\det(2aA_1 + bA_2)$$
$$= -\left(b + 2a\lambda\psi(\rho)\right)\left[2a\lambda\psi(\rho)\left(2\psi'(\rho)^2 - \psi''(\rho)\psi(\rho)\right) + \psi'(\rho)^2\left(b + 2a\lambda\psi(\rho)\right)\right].$$

The occurring derivatives of ψ are

$$\psi'(\rho) = \rho\sinh\rho \quad \text{and} \quad \psi''(\rho) = \rho\cosh\rho + \sinh\rho\,.$$

Thus, ψ is strictly increasing in ρ and positive for $\rho > 0$. So, for ρ sufficiently large[5] holds

$$0 > b > -2a\lambda\psi(\rho).$$

Moreover, we have that

$$2\psi'(\rho)^2 - \psi''(\rho)\psi(\rho) = \rho^2 \sinh^2\rho + \sinh^2\rho - \rho^2 > 0$$

for $\rho > 0$ and that this expression is also monotonically increasing in ρ. These observations imply that

$$\det(2aA_1 + bA_2) < 0$$

for ρ sufficiently large. Therefore, $2aA_1 + bA_2$ is indefinite.

The spectrum of the matrix αA_3 is obviously given by

$$\sigma(A_3) = \{0, 8\pi\alpha\}.$$

Choosing α sufficiently small and ρ as above, it follows that the Hessian $\mathcal{H}J_\alpha(\lambda, \rho) = 2aA_1 + bA_2 + \alpha A_3$ remains indefinite under the small perturbation αA_3, see [**Tao12**] for details on eigenvalues of sums of matrices. We conclude that the functional J_α is non-convex in general.

3.3.1. Existence, Stability and Regularization Property. Using similar techniques as in Section 3.1, we show in the following that the minimization problem (3.11) has a solution, which depends continuously on the data. Moreover, we see that the regularization property also holds for star-shaped domains.

Theorem 3.12 (Existence). *For any $\alpha > 0$ and any $g \in \mathcal{Y}$ there exists a solution $(\lambda^*, r^*, m^*) \in \Lambda \times \mathcal{R}$ of problem (3.11), that is,*

$$J_\alpha(\lambda^*, r^*, m^*) \leq J_\alpha(\lambda, r, m) \quad \text{for all } (\lambda, r, m) \in \Lambda \times \mathcal{R}.$$

PROOF. Let $\{(\lambda^n, r^n, m^n)\}_{n \in \mathbb{N}_0}$ be a minimizing sequence that monotonically decreases in J_α. The aim is to find a subsequence of this minimizing sequence that converges to a minimizer of J_α. The crucial part consists of constructing a link between Cauchy sequences of characteristic functions of star-shaped domains and Cauchy sequences of their parameterizations. This builds the basis for a compactness result in the variable r.

As the domains X_i are compact, there exists a tuple of points $m^* = (m_1^*, \ldots, m_I^*) \in \prod X_i$ and a subsequence $\{m^{n_k}\}_k \subset \prod X_i$ such that

$$m_i^{n_k} \to m_i^* \quad \text{as } k \to \infty, \quad i = 1, \ldots, I.$$

---

[5]We assume that the overall domain $B_R(0)$ is large enough, so that this choice for ρ is possible. Though both constants a and b depend on R, choosing a larger R does not cause any problems, since the constant a increases faster in R than $-b$.

By G^{n_k} we denote the tuple of domains parameterized by (r^{n_k}, m^{n_k}). As in the proof of Theorem 3.1, there exists a subsequence of $\{G^{n_k}\}$, which we again denote by $\{G^{n_k}\}$, converging to a tuple of measurable sets G^* in the sense that

$$\chi_{G_i^{n_k}} \to \chi_{G_i^*} \quad \text{in } L^1 \text{ as } k \to \infty, \quad i = 1, \ldots, I.$$

Let us consider the tuple of domains $\widetilde{G}^{n_k}$ parameterized by (r^{n_k}, m^*). We remark that $\widetilde{G}_i^{n_k}$ might be no subset of X_i, since the midpoint is changed into m^*. The following connection between G^{n_k} and $\widetilde{G}^{n_k}$ holds:

$$\chi_{\widetilde{G}_i^{n_k}} = \chi_{G_i^{n_k}}(\,\cdot\, + m_i^{n_k} - m_i^*), \quad i = 1, \ldots, I.$$

From the dominated convergence theorem, see e.g. [**Lan93**], follows that

$$\chi_{\widetilde{G}_i^{n_k}} \to \chi_{G_i^*} \quad \text{in } L^1 \text{ as } k \to \infty, \quad i = 1, \ldots, I.$$

For elements $\widetilde{G}_i^{n_k}$ and $\widetilde{G}_i^{n_l}$ we have the key relation

$$
\begin{aligned}
\int_X |\chi_{\widetilde{G}_i^{n_k}} - \chi_{\widetilde{G}_i^{n_l}}| \, \mathrm{d}x &= \int_{\widetilde{G}_i^{n_k} \triangle \widetilde{G}_i^{n_l}} 1 \, \mathrm{d}x \\
&= \int_{S^{d-1}} \int_{\min\{r_i^{n_k}, r_i^{n_l}\}}^{\max\{r_i^{n_k}, r_i^{n_l}\}} \rho^{d-1} \, \mathrm{d}\rho \, \mathrm{d}\theta \qquad (3.17) \\
&= \frac{1}{d} \int_{S^{d-1}} |(r_i^{n_k})^d - (r_i^{n_l})^d| \, \mathrm{d}\theta.
\end{aligned}
$$

Since the sequence $\{\widetilde{G}_i^{n_k}\}_k$ is convergent, it is especially a Cauchy sequence. The identity (3.17) reveals that $\{(r_i^{n_k})^d\}$ is a Cauchy sequence in L^1 as well, therefore convergent. We denote its limit by $\widetilde{r}_i \in L^1$ and observe $\widetilde{r}_i \geq 0$ almost everywhere, as $\{(r_i^n, m_i^n)\} \subset \mathcal{R}_i$. The L^1 convergence implies pointwise convergence almost everywhere, that is,

$$r_i^{n_k}(\theta) \to \widetilde{r}_i^{1/d}(\theta) \quad \text{as } k \to \infty \text{ for almost every } \theta \in S^{d-1}.$$

By Hölder's inequality,

$$\int_{S^{d-1}} |r_i^{n_k} - \widetilde{r}_i^{1/d}| \, \mathrm{d}\theta \leq \mathrm{Vol}(S^{d-1})^{1/d'} \left(\int_{S^{d-1}} |r_i^{n_k} - \widetilde{r}_i^{1/d}|^d \, \mathrm{d}\theta \right)^{1/d}$$

with $1/d + 1/d' = 1$. As

$$|r_i^{n_k} - \widetilde{r}_i^{1/d}|^d = \begin{cases} (r_i^{n_k})^2 - 2\widetilde{r}_i^{1/2} r_i^{n_k} + \widetilde{r}_i, & d = 2, \\ |(r_i^{n_k})^3 - 2\widetilde{r}_i^{1/3}(r_i^{n_k})^2 + 2\widetilde{r}_i^{2/3} r_i^{n_k} - \widetilde{r}_i|, & d = 3, \end{cases}$$

and $0 \leq r_i^{n_k} \leq \mathrm{diam}(X_i)$, the dominated convergence theorem yields

$$\int_{S^{d-1}} |r_i^{n_k} - \widetilde{r}_i^{1/d}| \, \mathrm{d}\theta \to 0 \quad \text{as } k \to \infty \, .$$

Let now $G_{r_i^*}$ be the domain parameterized by $r_i^* = \widetilde{r}_i^{1/d}$ and m_i^*. Then,

$$\frac{1}{d} \int_{S^{d-1}} |(r_i^{n_k})^d - (r_i^*)^d| \, \mathrm{d}\theta = \int_X |\chi_{\widetilde{G}_i^{n_k}} - \chi_{G_{r_i^*}}| \, \mathrm{d}x \, ,$$

which finally implies

$$\chi_{G_{r_i^*}} = \chi_{G_i^*} \, ,$$

since the limit is unique. Moreover, $(r_i^*, m_i^*) \in \mathcal{R}_i$ holds, as it is the limit of $\{(r_i^{n_k}, m_i^{n_k})\} \subset \mathcal{R}_i$ and as the set $\mathcal{R}_i$ is closed in L^1.

Due to the compactness of Λ, there exists a $\lambda^* \in \Lambda$ and a subsequence of $\{\lambda^{n_k}\}_k$, again denoted by $\{\lambda^{n_k}\}_k$, converging to λ^* as $k \to \infty$. In the same manner as in the proof of Theorem 3.1 follows that

$$J_\alpha(\lambda^*, r^*, m^*) \leq \liminf_{k \to \infty} J_\alpha(\lambda^{n_k}, r^{n_k}, m^{n_k}) = \liminf_{k \to \infty} J_\alpha(\lambda^{n_k}, G^{n_k}) \, .$$

Consequently, (λ^*, r^*, m^*) solves the minimization problem (3.11).   □

Combining the techniques of the last proof with the stability and regularization results of Section 3.1, we receive analogous results for star-shaped domains. Since the proofs are straightforward, we omit them.

Theorem 3.13 (Stability). *Let $g^n \to g$ in $\mathcal{Y}$ and denote by J_α^n the functional J_α with g substituted by g^n. Then, the sequence of minimizers (λ^n, r^n, m^n) of J_α^n over $\Lambda \times \mathcal{R}$ possesses a subsequence converging to a minimizer of J_α over $\Lambda \times \mathcal{R}$ in $\mathbb{R}^I \times \left(L^1(S^{d-1})\right)^I \times \mathbb{R}^I$.*

Furthermore, every convergent subsequence of $\{(\lambda^n, r^n, m^n)\}_n$ converges in $\mathbb{R}^I \times \left(L^1(S^{d-1})\right)^I \times \mathbb{R}^I$ to a minimizer of J_α.

Theorem 3.14 (Regularization Property). *Let g be given such that there exist an intensity vector $\widehat{\lambda} \in \Lambda$ and an I-tuple of star-shaped domains $\widehat{G}$ with parameterization $(\widehat{r}, \widehat{m}) \in \mathcal{R}$ satisfying $F(\widehat{\lambda}, \widehat{G}) = F(\widehat{\lambda}, \widehat{r}, \widehat{m}) = g$. Moreover, let $\{\delta_n\}_n$ be a positive null sequence and let $\{g_n\}_n$ be such that*

$$\|g_n - g\|_{\mathcal{Y}} \leq \delta_n \, .$$

Furthermore, let $\delta \mapsto \alpha(\delta)$ be a regularization parameter choice rule satisfying

$$\alpha(\delta) \to 0 \quad and \quad \frac{\delta^p}{\alpha(\delta)} \to 0 \quad as \, \delta \to 0 \, ,$$

where p is the exponent of the residual term in J_α. Then the sequence $\{(\lambda^n, r^n, m^n)\}$ of minimizers of $J^n_{\alpha(\delta_n)}$ over $\Lambda \times \mathcal{R}$ possesses a subsequence converging in $\mathbb{R}^I \times \left(L^1(S^{d-1})\right)^I \times \mathbb{R}^I$ to a solution (λ^+, r^+, m^+) of the unregularized problem 2.12 with

$$r^+ \in \arg\min\{\mathrm{Per}(r)\colon r \in \mathcal{R}_{\mathrm{sol}}\}. \tag{3.18}$$

Herein,

$$\mathcal{R}_{\mathrm{sol}} = \{r\colon \exists m \in \prod X_i, \lambda \in \Lambda \ s.t. \ (r, m) \in \mathcal{R}, F(\lambda, r, m) = g\}.$$

Moreover, every convergent subsequence of $\{(\lambda^n, r^n, m^n)\}_n$ converges in $\mathbb{R}^I \times \left(L^1(S^{d-1})\right)^I \times \mathbb{R}^I$ to a solution $(\lambda^\dagger, r^\dagger, m^\dagger)$ of Problem 2.12 meeting (3.18).

3.3.2. Approximation by Smooth Parameterizations.

Similar to Section 3.2 we develop an approximate variational principle for star-shaped domains. This result will be the basis for approximations to necessary conditions on minimizers of J_α and the justification to use optimization methods that converge to a critical point later in this work.

In the next lemma we see that smooth star-shaped domains are dense in the set of star-shaped domains with finite perimeter. This is an analogous result to Lemma 3.6.

Lemma 3.15. *Let $p \in [1, \infty[$ and $m \in \mathbb{R}^d$. Moreover, let $\rho \in L^p(S^{d-1})$ with $0 \le \rho \le \rho_{\max}$ a.e. such that the star-shaped domain Γ parameterized by (ρ, m) has finite perimeter. Then there exists a sequence $\{\rho^n\}_n \subset C^\infty(S^{d-1})$ with*

$$\|\rho^n - \rho\|_{L^p} \to 0 \quad \text{and} \quad \mathrm{Per}(\rho^n) \to \mathrm{Per}(\rho) \quad \text{as } n \to \infty.$$

PROOF. We recall that the perimeter of Γ is given by, cf. [**Giu84**],

$$\mathrm{Per}(\Gamma) = |D\chi_\Gamma| = \sup\left\{\int_{\mathbb{R}^d} \chi_\Gamma \mathrm{div}\varphi \, \mathrm{d}x\colon \varphi \in C^1(\mathbb{R}^d, \mathbb{R}^d), \|\varphi\|_\infty \le 1\right\}.$$

Using polar coordinates, we observe

$$\mathrm{Per}(\Gamma) \ge \int_{S^{d-1}} \int_0^{\rho(\theta)} \mathrm{div}\varphi(s, \theta) s^{d-1} \, \mathrm{d}s \, \mathrm{d}\theta$$

for any $\varphi \in C^1(\mathbb{R}^d, \mathbb{R}^d)$ with $\|\varphi\|_\infty \le 1$. Since $C^\infty(S^{d-1})$ is dense in $L^p(S^{d-1})$, there exists a uniformly bounded sequence $\{\rho^n\}_n \subset C^\infty(S^{d-1})$ such that

$$\|\rho^n - \rho\|_{L^p} \to 0 \quad \text{as } n \to \infty.$$

Let Γ^n be the domain parameterized by (ρ^n, m). By ν^n we denote the unit outward normal of Γ^n and $\varphi^n \in C^1(\mathbb{R}^d, \mathbb{R}^d)$ is an extension of ν^n

satisfying $\|\varphi^n\|_\infty \leq 1$. Applying first the dominated convergence theorem and then Gauß's theorem, we deduce that

$$
\begin{aligned}
\operatorname{Per}(\Gamma) &\geq \lim_{n\to\infty} \int_{S^{d-1}} \int_0^{\rho^n(\theta)} \operatorname{div}\varphi^n(s,\theta) s^{d-1} \,\mathrm{d}s\,\mathrm{d}\theta \\
&= \lim_{n\to\infty} \int_{\Gamma^n} \operatorname{div}\varphi^n(x)\,\mathrm{d}x = \lim_{n\to\infty} \int_{\partial\Gamma^n} \varphi^n \cdot \nu^n \,\mathrm{d}\mu \\
&= \lim_{n\to\infty} \mathcal{H}^{d-1}(\partial\Gamma^n) = \lim_{n\to\infty} \operatorname{Per}(\Gamma^n).
\end{aligned} \tag{3.19}
$$

Please note that the last equation holds true, because Γ^n is a smooth domain.

Like in the proof of Theorem 3.12, we see that

$$
\chi_{\Gamma^n} \to \chi_\Gamma \quad \text{in } L^1(\mathbb{R}^d) \text{ as } n \to \infty.
$$

In view of (3.19) and the lower semicontinuity of the perimeter, that is, $\operatorname{Per}(\Gamma) \leq \liminf_{n\to\infty} \operatorname{Per}(\Gamma^n)$, we conclude that

$$
\operatorname{Per}(\rho^n) \to \operatorname{Per}(\rho) \quad \text{as } n \to \infty.
$$

$\square$

The approximate variational principle assumes the following form in the star-shaped framework:

Theorem 3.16 (Approximate Variational Principle). *Let $\mathcal{U}$ be a Banach space with $C^\infty(S^{d-1})^I \subset \mathcal{U} \subset C^2(S^{d-1})^I$ and let $(\lambda^*, r^*, m^*) \in \Lambda \times \mathcal{R}$ be a minimizer of J_α. Additionally, let $\varepsilon > 0$ and $(\widetilde{r}^\varepsilon, m^*) \in (\mathcal{U} \times \mathbb{R}^{dI}) \cap \mathcal{R}$ such that*

$$
J_\alpha(\lambda^*, \widetilde{r}^\varepsilon, m^*) < J_\alpha(\lambda^*, r^*, m^*) + \varepsilon. \tag{3.20}
$$

Assume that for an $R > 0$ the inclusion

$$
B_R(\widetilde{r}^\varepsilon, m^*) \subset \mathcal{R}
$$

holds, where $B_R(\widetilde{r}^\varepsilon, m^*)$ is the closed ball in $\mathcal{U} \times \mathbb{R}^{dI}$ with radius R centered at $(\widetilde{r}^\varepsilon, m^*)$.

Then for every $\gamma \in \,]0, R[$ there exist a point $(r^\varepsilon, m^\varepsilon) \in (\mathcal{U} \times \mathbb{R}^{dI}) \cap \mathcal{R}$ and a $\lambda^\varepsilon \in \Lambda$ with

$$
\|(\lambda^\varepsilon - \lambda^*, r^\varepsilon - \widetilde{r}^\varepsilon, m^\varepsilon - m^*)\| \leq \gamma \tag{3.21}
$$

such that

$$
J_\alpha(\lambda^\varepsilon, r^\varepsilon, m^\varepsilon) \leq J_\alpha(\lambda^*, \widetilde{r}^\varepsilon, m^*), \tag{3.22}
$$

$$
J_\alpha(\lambda^\varepsilon, r^\varepsilon, m^\varepsilon) - \frac{\varepsilon}{\gamma}\|(h_\lambda, h_r, h_m)\| < J_\alpha(\lambda^\varepsilon + h_\lambda, r^\varepsilon + h_r, m^\varepsilon + h_m) \tag{3.23}
$$

for all $\lambda^\varepsilon + h_\lambda \in \Lambda \setminus \{\lambda^\varepsilon\}$ and $(r^\varepsilon + h_r, m^\varepsilon + h_m) \in B_R(\widetilde{r}^\varepsilon, m^*) \setminus \{(r^\varepsilon, m^\varepsilon)\}$. The norm $\| \cdot \|$, occurring in (3.21) and (3.23), is the one of the space $\mathbb{R}^I \times \mathcal{U} \times \mathbb{R}^{dI}$.

PROOF. The assertion is an immediate consequence of Ekeland's ε-variational principle [**Eke74**, Theorem 1.1] applied in $\Lambda \times B_R(\widetilde{r}^\varepsilon, m^*)$. □

We note, analogous to Remark 3.10, that for all $\varepsilon > 0$ we always find a pair $(\widetilde{r}^\varepsilon, m^*) \in (\mathcal{U} \times \mathbb{R}^{dI}) \cap \mathcal{R}$ satisfying the inequality (3.20). The reason for this is again the density result in Lemma 3.15 and the continuity of the norm term in J_α.

In the next chapter and Chapter 6 we derive the domain derivative of the forward operator F in the diffusion and transport model, respectively. Based on the calculated derivative and on Theorem 3.16, we elaborate estimates on the derivative of J_α near the star-shaped minimizer in the mentioned chapters.

Part II

Diffusion Approximation based Bioluminescence Tomography

CHAPTER 4

Domain Derivative of the DA-based Forward Operator

We turn now to the model specific analysis. Since the diffusion model is simpler and the theory is more complete in this framework, we start with this model in this part of the thesis. A crucial gap to extend the theory developed in the last chapter builds the domain derivative of the forward operator. We derive it in Section 4.1 for DA-based BLT. As the domain derivative is known for a broad class of inverse problems based on second-order elliptic, see e.g. [**Het99**], we only present the derivation for a special case in order to gain a better understanding. Our calculations are inspired by an idea used in level set approaches for inverse problems in [**San96, Dor02**]. For a detailed derivation in a broader framework we refer to [**Het99**]. Given the domain derivative of F, the domain derivative of J_α is easily obtained. Moreover, the approximate variational principles can be specified further. These consequences are described in Section 4.2.

In this part we need to refine the assumptions made in Section 2.2.2. We assume that the domain X has sufficiently smooth boundary and that $D, \sigma_a \in C^1(X)$ are bounded away from zero by constants D_0 and σ_0, respectively: $0 < D_0 \leq D$ and $0 < \sigma_0 \leq \sigma_a$ almost everywhere in X.

Let us recall a few definitions for the sake of convenience. The linear forward operator of DA-based BLT is given by

$$A\colon L^2(X) \to L^2(\partial X) = \mathcal{Y}, \quad q \mapsto u|_{\partial X},$$

compare equation (2.30). Herein, u is the weak solution of the boundary value problem (2.29), that is,

$$-\operatorname{div}\left(D\nabla u\right)+\sigma_a u = q \quad \text{in } X, \quad u + 2D\frac{\partial u}{\partial \nu} = 0 \quad \text{on } \partial X. \qquad (4.1)$$

Using the *a priori* knowledge of piecewise constant sources, discussed in Section 2.3, we obtain the nonlinear forward operator

$$F\colon \Lambda \times \mathcal{L} \to \mathcal{Y}, \quad (\lambda, G) \mapsto \sum_{i=1}^{I} \lambda_i A\chi_{G_i}, \qquad (4.2)$$

which is definition (2.35).

4.1. Derivation of the Domain Derivative of F

In this section we derive the domain derivative of F about a smooth shape $G \in \mathcal{G}$, i.e., about a shape with C^2 boundary. As mentioned in the introduction above, we present the derivation for a special case only, namely for connected C^2 domains. Motivated by this, we state the general result afterwards.

4.1.1. The Domain Derivative of F about a Domain.
Let $\Gamma \subset X$ be a connected domain with C^2 boundary and let $\lambda \in \Lambda$ be fixed in this section. As in Subsection 3.2.1, we define for $h \in C_0^1(X, \mathbb{R}^d)$ the perturbed domain by

$$\Gamma_h = \{x + h(x)\colon x \in \Gamma\},$$

which is again a connected subdomain of X for h small enough. The aim is to find the domain derivative of F about Γ, i.e., an operator $\partial_\Gamma F(\lambda, \Gamma) \in \mathcal{L}(C_0^1, \mathcal{Y})$ such that

$$\|F(\lambda, \Gamma_h) - F(\lambda, \Gamma) - \partial_\Gamma F(\lambda, \Gamma)h\|_{\mathcal{Y}} = o\left(\|h\|_{C^1}\right).$$

To keep the notation precise, we set the number of sources $I = 1$ in this analysis.

Inspired by [**San96**], where the effect of small changes in the level set function on the corresponding characteristic function is calculated formally, we derive the domain derivative of the operator

$$Q\colon \mathcal{L} \to \widetilde{H}^{-1}(X), \quad Q(G) = \lambda\chi_G, \qquad (4.3)$$

about Γ in a first step. Herein, $\widetilde{H}^{-1}(X)$ denotes again the dual space of $H^1(X)$. Since the linear forward operator A is also bounded from $\widetilde{H}^{-1}(X)$ to $\mathcal{Y}$, the domain derivative of F is then an immediate consequence.

We set $q_h = \lambda\chi_{\Gamma_h}$. In addition, let $v \in H^1(X)$ be a test function. Then,

$$\langle q_h - q, v\rangle_{L^2(X)} = \int_X (q_h - q)v \,\mathrm{d}x = \int_{\Gamma_h \Delta \Gamma} \Delta q_h v \,\mathrm{d}x \qquad (4.4)$$

with the symmetric difference $\Gamma_h \Delta \Gamma = (\Gamma_h \setminus \Gamma) \cup (\Gamma \setminus \Gamma_h)$ and with

$$\Delta q_h(x) = \begin{cases} \lambda, & x \in \Gamma_h \setminus \Gamma, \\ -\lambda, & x \in \Gamma \setminus \Gamma_h, \\ 0, & \text{otherwise}. \end{cases}$$

Recombining the findings in [**BG88**, Chapter 6], we have the following change of variables result: There exist functions $\psi_1, \psi_2 \in C(\partial \Gamma)$ such that

$$\int_{\Gamma_h \Delta \Gamma} f(x)\, \mathrm{d}x = \int_{\partial \Gamma} \int_{\min\{0, h_\nu(y)\}}^{\max\{h_\nu(y), 0\}} f\big(y + t\nu(y)\big) \Psi\big(y, t\nu(y)\big)\, \mathrm{d}t\, \mathrm{d}\mu(y)$$

for $f \in L^1(\Gamma_h \Delta \Gamma)$, where ν is the outer unit normal of Γ, $h_\nu = h \cdot \nu$ and

$$\Psi\big(y, t\nu(y)\big) = 1 + t\psi_1(y) + t^2 \psi_2(y). \tag{4.5}$$

We apply this change of variables to equation (4.4) and obtain

$$\begin{aligned} \langle q_h - q, v \rangle_{L^2(X)} &= \int_{\partial \Gamma} \Big(\lambda h_\nu + o\big(\|h\|_{C^1}\big)\Big) v\, \mathrm{d}\mu \\ &= \int_{\partial \Gamma} \lambda h_\nu v\, \mathrm{d}\mu + \|v|_{\partial \Gamma}\|_{L^1(\partial \Gamma)} o\big(\|h\|_{C^1}\big) \\ &= \langle \lambda h_\nu \delta_{\partial \Gamma}, v \rangle_{L^2(X)} + \|v|_{\partial \Gamma}\|_{L^1(\partial \Gamma)} o\big(\|h\|_{C^1}\big). \end{aligned} \tag{4.6}$$

Herein, $\delta_{\partial \Gamma}$ is the trace operator mapping a function to its trace on $\partial \Gamma$, which can also be interpreted as delta distribution on $\partial \Gamma$. In the last identity of (4.6) we use the fact that the dual form on $H^1(X) \times \widetilde{H}^{-1}(X)$ is the continuous extension of the inner product in $L^2(X)$ to the dual pairing, see e.g. [**Wlo87**]. Taking this into account again as well as the validity of equation (4.6) for every test function $v \in H^1(X)$, we get the estimate

$$\|q_h - q - \lambda h_\nu \delta_{\partial \Gamma}\|_{\widetilde{H}^{-1}} = o\big(\|h\|_{C^1}\big). \tag{4.7}$$

Consequently, the distribution $\lambda h_\nu \delta_{\partial \Gamma}$ is the domain derivative of Q about Γ in direction h, that is,

$$Q'(\Gamma)h = \lambda h_\nu \delta_{\partial \Gamma}. \tag{4.8}$$

As mentioned above, the linear forward operator A is bounded from $\widetilde{H}^{-1}(X)$ to $\mathcal{Y}$. Applying A to the sum of distributions in (4.7) and recalling the definition of F in (4.2), we find immediately that

$$\|F(\lambda, \Gamma_h) - F(\lambda, \Gamma) - \lambda A(h_\nu \delta_{\partial \Gamma})\|_{\mathcal{Y}} = o\big(\|h\|_{C^1}\big).$$

Thus, $\lambda A(h_\nu \delta_{\partial \Gamma})$ is the domain derivative of $F(\lambda, \cdot)$ about Γ in direction h. We specify it further. Let $u' \in H^1(X)$ be the weak solution of the diffusion equation (4.1) with source term $\lambda h_\nu \delta_{\partial\Gamma}$, i.e., solution of

$$\int_X (D\nabla u' \cdot \nabla v + \sigma_a u' v)\, \mathrm{d}x + \frac{1}{2}\int_{\partial X} u'v\, \mathrm{d}\mu = \lambda \int_{\partial\Gamma} h_\nu v\, \mathrm{d}\mu \qquad (4.9)$$

for all $v \in H^1(X)$. This is exactly the weak formulation of the transmission boundary value problem

$$-\mathrm{div}(D\nabla u') + \mu u' = 0 \quad \text{in } X \setminus \partial\Gamma\,,$$

$$[u']_\pm = 0 \quad \text{on } \partial\Gamma\,,$$

$$\left[D\frac{\partial u'}{\partial \nu}\right]_\pm = -\lambda h_\nu \quad \text{on } \partial\Gamma\,, \qquad (4.10)$$

$$2D\frac{\partial u'}{\partial \nu} + u' = 0 \quad \text{on } \partial X\,.$$

Herein, the symbol $[f]_\pm$ denotes the jump of a function f at the interface $\partial\Gamma$, that is,

$$[f]_\pm = f|_+ - f|_-\,,$$

where the symbols $|_+$ and $|_-$ indicate the trace of f approaching $\partial\Gamma$ from the exterior $X \setminus \overline{\Gamma}$ and the interior Γ, respectively. By the definition of A it is clear that $u'|_{\partial X} = \lambda A(h_\nu \delta_{\partial\Gamma})$. We conclude that

$$\partial_\Gamma F(\lambda, \Gamma)h = \lambda A(h_\nu \delta_{\partial\Gamma}) = u'|_{\partial X}\,. \qquad (4.11)$$

This derivation can be naturally extended to domains Γ that are a finite union of disjoint connected domains. However, the argumentation might fail for general C^2 shapes. The problem arises when Γ is a union of infinitely many disjoint connected domains. It is not sure if the functions ψ_1 and ψ_2 of equation (4.5) are uniformly bounded on $\partial\Gamma$ in this case. Therefore, we have to consider a different approach in the next subsection to cover the general case.

4.1.2. The Domain Derivative of F: General Case.

In a different way from our presentation in the last subsection, the domain derivative can also be derived by applying a change of variables to the weak formulation of the diffusion equation with source term q_h and by estimating the difference of the weak forms cleverly. This approach is performed in [**HR96**] for an inverse source problem in potential theory and in [**Het99**] for a general class of inverse problems based on second-order elliptic differential equations.

The derivation in these works leads to exactly the same result as obtained in the previous subsection for connected domains Γ, compare equation (4.11). However, the calculations based on the change of variables work also for infinitely many sources, i.e., extend to the general case.

Our statement on the domain derivative of F about general C^2 shapes is therefore adopted from [**Het99**]. We refer to this work for the proof.

Theorem 4.1. *The derivative of the forward operator F defined in* (4.2) *with respect to the ith shape G_i in direction $h \in C_0^2(X_i, \mathbb{R}^d)$ about $(\lambda, G) \in \Lambda \times \mathcal{G}$ is given by*

$$\partial_{G_i} F(\lambda, G) h = u_i'|_{\partial X} ,$$

where $u_i' \in H^1(X)$ is the solution of the transmission boundary value problem (4.10) *with Γ replaced by G_i.*

PROOF. See [**Het99**, Theorem 2.9].   □

4.2. Consequences for the Minimization Problem

Now having the domain derivative of the forward operator at hand, we can calculate the derivative of the minimization functional J_α with respect to both arguments. Based on this, we specify some results found in the general analysis of Chapter 3. These findings have been published before in [**KR12**].

4.2.1. The Derivative of the Minimization Functional J_α.

The forward operator F, see (4.2), does not only depend on the shape variable G but also on the intensity variable λ. The dependency is only linear, though. Thus, the partial Fréchet derivative with respect to the intensity in direction $k \in \mathbb{R}^I$ about $(\lambda, G) \in \Lambda \times \mathcal{G}$ is given by

$$\partial_\lambda F(\lambda, G) k = \sum_{i=1}^{I} k_i A \chi_{G_i} .$$

Combining this with the domain derivative of F obtained above and of the perimeter functional Per stated in Lemma 3.7, we are able to differentiate the regularization functional J_α in the diffusive framework. For convenience we recall the definition of J_α, compare (2.37):

$$J_\alpha(\lambda, G) = \frac{1}{2} \|F(\lambda, G) - g\|_{\mathcal{Y}}^2 + \alpha \text{Per}(G) .$$

Theorem 4.2 (Derivative of J_α in DA-based BLT). *The derivative of the functional J_α about $(\lambda, G) \in \Lambda \times \mathcal{G}$ is given by*

$$J'_\alpha(\lambda, G)(k, h) = \sum_{i=1}^{I} \left[\langle u|_{\partial X} - g, k_i v_i|_{\partial X} + u'_i|_{\partial X} \rangle_{\mathcal{Y}} + \alpha \int_{\partial G_i} \mathrm{H}_{\partial G_i} h_{i,\nu} \, d\mu \right]$$

for $k \in \mathbb{R}^I$ and $h \in \prod_{i=1}^{I} C_0^2(X_i, \mathbb{R}^d)$, where $u|_{\partial X} = A \sum_{i=1}^{I} \lambda_i \chi_{G_i}$ and $v_i|_{\partial X} = A\chi_{G_i}$. The term u'_i is the solution of the transmission boundary value problem (4.10) *with λ, Γ and h_ν replaced by λ_i, G_i and $h_{i,\nu}$, respectively.*

PROOF. Elementary derivative computations, cf. [**AH05**, Section 5.3], lead to

$$J'_\alpha(\lambda, G)(k, h) = \partial_\lambda J_\alpha(\lambda, G)k + \partial_G J_\alpha(\lambda, G)h$$

$$= \langle F(\lambda, G) - g, \partial_\lambda F(\lambda, G)k + \partial_G F(\lambda, G)h \rangle_{\mathcal{Y}} + \alpha \partial_G \mathrm{Per}(G)h$$

$$= \sum_{i=1}^{I} \left[\langle F(\lambda, G) - g, \partial_{\lambda_i} F(\lambda, G)k_i + \partial_{G_i} F(\lambda, G)h_i \rangle_{\mathcal{Y}} + \alpha \partial_{G_i} \mathrm{Per}(G)h_i \right],$$

which readily yields the assertion.   □

4.2.2. The Approximate Variational Principle Revisited: General C^2 Shapes. In Subsection 3.2.2 we derived a quite general approximate variational principle. The main result is Theorem 3.9, which states roughly speaking: If (λ^*, G^*) is a minimizer of J_α and $G^\varepsilon \in \mathcal{G}$ is such that

$$J_\alpha(\lambda^*, G^\varepsilon) \leq J_\alpha(\lambda^*, G^*) + \varepsilon,$$

then we find for every sufficiently small positive number γ an intensity $\lambda^\varepsilon \in \Lambda$ and a perturbed shape G_v^ε that are near $(\lambda^*, G^\varepsilon)$ and that are non-increasing in J_α, i.e., that satisfy

$$\|(\lambda^\varepsilon - \lambda^*, v)\|_{\mathbb{R}^I \times \mathcal{V}} \leq \gamma \quad \text{and} \quad J_\alpha(\lambda^\varepsilon, G_v^\varepsilon) \leq J_\alpha(\lambda^*, G^\varepsilon).$$

Additionally, the estimate

$$J_\alpha(\lambda^\varepsilon, G_v^\varepsilon) - \frac{\varepsilon}{\gamma} \|(k, h)\|_{\mathbb{R}^I \times \mathcal{V}} < J_\alpha(\lambda^\varepsilon + k, G_{v+h}^\varepsilon) \qquad (4.12)$$

holds for all h, k sufficiently small. Herein, $\mathcal{V}$ is a Banach space with $\mathcal{V} \subset \prod_{i=1}^{I} C_0^2(X_i, \mathbb{R}^d)$ and $\|v\|_{C^2} \leq C\|v\|_{\mathcal{V}}$ for a constant $C > 0$.

The estimate (4.12) together with the differentiability of J_α yields an estimate on the norm of $J'_\alpha(\lambda, G_v^\varepsilon)$, which we present in the following corollary to Theorem 3.9. It is an adaption of Ekeland's ε-variational principle for Fréchet differentiable functionals, cf. e.g. [**Eke74**, Theorem 2.2], to the domain differentiable functional J_α.

Corollary 4.3. *Let the assumptions of Theorem 3.9 be satisfied and in addition λ^* be an inner point of Λ. Moreover, let there exist a constant $\widetilde{C} \geq 1$ such that $\|h\|_{\mathcal{V}} \leq \widetilde{C}\|h \circ (I + v)^{-1}\|_{\mathcal{V}}$ for all $h \in \mathcal{V}$. Then,*

$$\|J'_\alpha(\lambda^\varepsilon, G^\varepsilon_v)\|_{\mathbb{R}^I \times \mathcal{V} \to \mathbb{R}} \leq \widetilde{C}\frac{\varepsilon}{\gamma}. \tag{4.13}$$

PROOF. From Theorem 3.9 we know that estimate (4.12) holds for all $\lambda^\varepsilon + k \in \Lambda \setminus \{\lambda^\varepsilon\}$ and $v + h \in \mathcal{V} \setminus \{v\}$ with $\|v + h\|_{\mathcal{V}} \leq \frac{1}{2C}$. From this estimate we derive (4.13). We set $\widetilde{h} = h \circ (\mathrm{id} + v)^{-1}$ and observe the identity $G_{v+h} = (G_v)_{\widetilde{h}}$. The differentiability of J_α about $(\lambda^\varepsilon, G^\varepsilon_v)$ yields that

$$J_\alpha\big(\lambda^\varepsilon + tk, G^\varepsilon_{v+th}\big) - J_\alpha(\lambda^\varepsilon, G^\varepsilon_v) = J'_\alpha(\lambda^\varepsilon, G^\varepsilon_v)t(k, \widetilde{h}) + o\big(\|t(k, \widetilde{h})\|_{\mathbb{R}^I \times C^2}\big).$$

Letting $t \to 0$ and taking (4.12) into account, we obtain

$$-\frac{\varepsilon}{\gamma}\|(k, h)\|_{\mathbb{R}^I \times \mathcal{V}} \leq J'_\alpha(\lambda^\varepsilon, G^\varepsilon_v)(k, \widetilde{h})$$

for all $(k, h) \in \mathbb{R}^I \times \mathcal{V}$ and with $\widetilde{h} = h \circ (\mathrm{id} + v)^{-1}$. Hence,

$$|J'_\alpha(\lambda^\varepsilon, G^\varepsilon_v)(k, \widetilde{h})| \leq \frac{\varepsilon}{\gamma}\|(k, h)\|_{\mathbb{R}^I \times \mathcal{V}}.$$

The proof is completed dividing by $\|(k, \widetilde{h})\|_{\mathbb{R}^I \times \mathcal{V}}$ and recalling the definition of the constant $\widetilde{C}$. $\qquad\square$

Remark 4.4. For the space $\prod C^2(X_i, \mathbb{R}^3)$ we have

$$\|h\|_{C^2} \leq 2(1 + \gamma)^2\|h \circ (\mathrm{id} + v)^{-1}\|_{C^2},$$

where γ is the upper bound of the norm of v as defined in Theorem 3.9. Thus, the hypothesis of the previous corollary is satisfied with $\widetilde{C} = 2(1 + \gamma)^2$. That can be seen from applying the chain rule to $h = \widetilde{h} \circ (\mathrm{id} + v)$.

Remark 4.5. In contrast to the general result in Theorem 3.9, the additional assumption that each component of G^ε is a finite union of disjoint connected sets if $d = 3$ has not to be imposed to obtain the approximate variational principle in the diffusion model. In the DA-based framework the continuity of J_α in the geometric variable follows directly from the domain differentiability. Lemma 3.8 is not needed for this purpose, as opposed to Theorem 3.9.

Relying on the approximation result in Lemma 3.6, the estimate on the volume of the symmetric difference in Lemma 3.8 and the last corollary, we verify the existence of almost stationary C^2 shapes near the minimizer.

This can be interpreted as an approximation to the well-known necessary condition on a minimizer of J_α.

Theorem 4.6. *Let (λ^*, G^*) be a minimizer of J_α and λ^* an inner point of Λ. In case $d = 3$, assume that each component of G^* is a finite union of disjoint connected domains. Then for any $\varepsilon > 0$ sufficiently small we can find an intensity vector $\lambda^\varepsilon \in \Lambda$ and an I-tuple of C^2 sets $G^\varepsilon \in \mathcal{G}$ satisfying*

$$J_\alpha(\lambda^\varepsilon, G^\varepsilon) - J_\alpha(\lambda^*, G^*) \leq \varepsilon,$$

$$\sum_{i=1}^{I} \|\lambda_i^\varepsilon \chi_{G_i^\varepsilon} - \lambda_i^* \chi_{G_i^*}\|_{L^1} \leq \varepsilon,$$

$$\|J_\alpha'(\lambda^\varepsilon, G^\varepsilon)\|_{\mathbb{R}^I \times C^2 \to \mathbb{R}} \leq \varepsilon.$$

PROOF. Let $\varepsilon_1 > 0$. By Lemma 3.6 there exists $\widetilde{G}^\varepsilon \in \mathcal{G}$ with

$$\sum_{i=1}^{I} \|\chi_{\widetilde{G}_i^\varepsilon} - \chi_{G_i^*}\|_{L^1} \leq \varepsilon_1 \quad \text{and} \quad |\mathrm{Per}(\widetilde{G}^\varepsilon) - \mathrm{Per}(G^*)| \leq \varepsilon_1.$$

In case $d = 3$, each component $\widetilde{G}_i^\varepsilon$ is a finite union of disjoint connected domains for ε_1 sufficiently small. Let N be the maximal number of disjoint connected domains. Due to the continuity of the norm term in J_α and due to the above inequalities we get

$$J_\alpha(\lambda^*, \widetilde{G}^\varepsilon) - J_\alpha(\lambda^*, G^*) \leq \varepsilon_2$$

for an $\varepsilon_2 > 0$ getting smaller with ε_1. Applying Theorem 3.9 and Corollary 4.3 with $\gamma = \sqrt{\varepsilon_2} =: \varepsilon_3$, we obtain a $\lambda^\varepsilon \in \Lambda$, a C^2 function h and the C^2 shape $G^\varepsilon = \widetilde{G}_h^\varepsilon$ fulfilling

$$J_\alpha(\lambda^\varepsilon, G^\varepsilon) - J_\alpha(\lambda^*, G^*) \leq \varepsilon_2,$$

$$\|(\lambda^\varepsilon - \lambda^*, h)\|_{\mathbb{R}^I \times C^2} \leq \varepsilon_3,$$

$$\|J_\alpha'(\lambda^\varepsilon, G^\varepsilon)\|_{\mathbb{R}^I \times C^2 \to \mathbb{R}} \leq \widetilde{C}\varepsilon_3.$$

Using Lemma 3.8 and setting $C_2 = 0$ and $C_3 = 8\pi IN/3$, we observe

$$\sum_{i=1}^{I} \|\chi_{\widetilde{G}_i^\varepsilon} - \chi_{G_i^\varepsilon}\|_{L^1} = \sum_{i=1}^{I} \|\chi_{\widetilde{G}_i^\varepsilon \Delta G_i^\varepsilon}\|_{L^1} \leq \big(\mathrm{Per}(\widetilde{G}^\varepsilon) + C_d \|h\|_\infty^2\big)\|h\|_\infty$$

$$\leq \big(\mathrm{Per}(G^*) + \varepsilon_1 + C_d \varepsilon_3^2\big)\varepsilon_3.$$

By the triangle inequality,

$$\sum_{i=1}^{I} \|\chi_{G_i^\varepsilon} - \chi_{G_i^*}\|_{L^1} \leq \big(\mathrm{Per}(G^*) + \varepsilon_1 + C_d \varepsilon_3^2\big)\varepsilon_3 + \varepsilon_1 =: \varepsilon_4.$$

Thus,

$$\sum_{i=1}^{I} \|\lambda_i^\varepsilon \chi_{G_i^\varepsilon} - \lambda_i^* \chi_{G_i^*}\|_{L^1} \leq \sum_{i=1}^{I} \left(|\lambda_i^\varepsilon| \|\chi_{G_i^\varepsilon} - \chi_{G_i^*}\|_{L^1} + |\lambda_i^\varepsilon - \lambda_i^*| \|\chi_{G_i^*}\|_{L^1} \right)$$

$$\leq \max_{i \in I} |\lambda_i^\varepsilon| \varepsilon_4 + \mathrm{Vol}(X)\varepsilon_3 \leq \mathrm{L}\varepsilon_4 + \mathrm{Vol}(X)\varepsilon_3$$

with $\mathrm{L} = \max\{|l| \mid l \in \bigcup_{i=1}^{I} \Lambda_i\}$. The right-hand side of the last estimate converges to 0 for $\varepsilon_1 \to 0$. Choosing now ε_1 sufficiently small shows the assertion. $\qquad\square$

Remark 4.7. The results of the previous theorem are not limited to C^2 shapes. For shapes with higher regularity a similar statement under the assumptions of Corollary 4.3 can be proven.

4.2.3. The Approximate Variational Principle Revisited: Star-shaped Domains. Analogous consequences of the approximate variational principle for star-shaped domains can be derived from the findings in Section 3.3.2. To do so, we proceed in a similar manner as in the last paragraph for general C^2 shapes.

Since with the parameterization of the boundary we have a linear structure at hand, the derivative with respect to the geometric variable, i.e., the parameterization, is just the usual Fréchet derivative. So, the analog to Corollary 4.3 in the star-shaped setting is a simple application of Ekeland's ε-variational principle for differentiable functionals [**Eke74**, Theorem 2.2].

Corollary 4.8. *Let the assumptions of Theorem 3.16 be satisfied. Moreover, let λ^* be an inner point of Λ. Then,*

$$\|J_\alpha'(\lambda^\varepsilon, r^\varepsilon, m^\varepsilon)\|_{\mathbb{R}^I \times \mathcal{U} \times \mathbb{R}^{dI} \to \mathbb{R}} \leq \frac{\varepsilon}{\gamma}$$

holds, using the notation of Theorem 3.16.

The approximation to the necessary condition of a minimizer is derived as above but using the corresponding results for star-shaped domains. We obtain the following existence result of almost stationary smooth parameterization near the optimal one.

Theorem 4.9. *Let $\mathcal{U}$ be a Banach space with $C^\infty(S^{d-1})^I \subset \mathcal{U} \subset C^2(S^{d-1})^I$ and $C \geq 1$ a constant satisfying $\|\cdot\|_{(L^1)^I} \leq C\|\cdot\|_{\mathcal{U}}$.*

If the minimizer (λ^*, r^*, m^*) of J_α is an interior point of $\Lambda \times \mathcal{R}$ with respect to the $\mathbb{R}^I \times (L^1)^I \times \mathbb{R}^{dI}$ metric, then for any $\varepsilon > 0$ sufficiently small *there exists a point* $(\lambda^\varepsilon, r^\varepsilon, m^\varepsilon) \in \Lambda \times \left((\mathcal{U} \times \mathbb{R}^{dI}) \cap \mathcal{R}\right)$ *with*

$$J_\alpha(\lambda^\varepsilon, r^\varepsilon, m^\varepsilon) - J_\alpha(\lambda^*, r^*, m^*) \leq \varepsilon,$$

$$\|(\lambda^\varepsilon, r^\varepsilon, m^\varepsilon) - (\lambda^*, r^*, m^*)\|_{\mathbb{R}^I \times (L^1)^I \times \mathbb{R}^{dI}} \leq \varepsilon,$$

$$\|J_\alpha'(\lambda^\varepsilon, r^\varepsilon, m^\varepsilon)\|_{\mathbb{R}^I \times \mathcal{U} \times \mathbb{R}^{dI} \to \mathbb{R}} \leq \varepsilon.$$

PROOF. We proceed similar to the proof of Theorem 4.6: By Lemma 3.15, we find for any $\varepsilon_1 > 0$ a tuple of functions $\tilde{r}^\varepsilon \in \mathcal{U}$ such that

$$\|\tilde{r}^\varepsilon - r^*\|_{(L^1)^I} \leq \varepsilon_1 \quad \text{and} \quad |\text{Per}(\tilde{r}^\varepsilon) - \text{Per}(r^*)| \leq \varepsilon_1.$$

Since the minimizer is an interior point, we have $(\tilde{r}^\varepsilon, m^*) \in \mathcal{R}$ for sufficiently small $\varepsilon_1 > 0$. Recalling (3.17), the boundedness of $\tilde{r}^\varepsilon$ and r^* as well as the continuity of the residual term in J_α, there exists an ε_2, which goes to zero when ε_1 does, with

$$J_\alpha(\lambda^*, \tilde{r}^\varepsilon, m^*) - J_\alpha(\lambda^*, r^*, m^*) \leq \varepsilon_2.$$

Applying now Theorem 3.16 and Corollary 4.8 with $\gamma = \sqrt{\varepsilon_2}$, we get a point $(\lambda^\varepsilon, r^\varepsilon, m^\varepsilon) \in \Lambda \times \left((\mathcal{U} \times \mathbb{R}^{dI}) \cap \mathcal{R}\right)$ satisfying

$$J_\alpha(\lambda^\varepsilon, r^\varepsilon, m^\varepsilon) - J_\alpha(\lambda^*, r^*, m^*) \leq \varepsilon_2,$$

$$\|(\lambda^\varepsilon, r^\varepsilon, m^\varepsilon) - (\lambda^*, \tilde{r}^\varepsilon, m^*)\|_{\mathbb{R}^I \times \mathcal{U} \times \mathbb{R}^{dI}} \leq \sqrt{\varepsilon_2},$$

$$\|J_\alpha'(\lambda^\varepsilon, r^\varepsilon, m^\varepsilon)\|_{\mathbb{R}^I \times \mathcal{U} \times \mathbb{R}^{dI} \to \mathbb{R}} \leq \sqrt{\varepsilon_2}.$$

Obviously, it follows that

$$\|(\lambda^\varepsilon, r^\varepsilon, m^\varepsilon) - (\lambda^*, r^*, m^*)\|_{\mathbb{R}^I \times (L^1)^I \times \mathbb{R}^{dI}} \leq C\sqrt{\varepsilon_2} + \varepsilon_1.$$

Choosing ε_1 sufficiently small shows the assertion.   □

We point out that the observation of the previous theorem is the justification to use optimization methods that converge to a critical point in the upcoming chapter.

CHAPTER 5

Numerical Experiments for DA-based Bioluminescence Tomography

After the analytical study of the DA-based BLT problem in the last chapters, we now consider the problem from a numerical point of view. In Section 5.1 we introduce the optimization methods that are used for solving the Problem 2.13. Several numerical experiments, all in two dimensions, are discussed in Section 5.2. We point out that the presented numerical schemes and implementation serve as proof of concept and to illustrate our theoretical findings. Improvements of both are certainly possible, but beyond the scope of this work. This chapter is a revision and an extension of the numerical part of [**KR12**].

5.1. Numerical Schemes

In this section we develop descent methods to minimize J_α for star-shaped domains. Since this functional is not differentiable with respect to general domains, we restrict ourselves to a dense subspace $\mathcal{U} \subset C^2(S^{d-1})^I$, where $\mathcal{U}$ is assumed to be a Hilbert space. In view of Theorem 4.9, there exist smooth almost stationary points in any neighborhood of a minimizer. Therefore, we expect that a descent method converging to a stationary point in $\Lambda \times \mathcal{U}$ also converges to a minimizer of J_α.

Further, we have to implement the constraints $\lambda \in \Lambda$ and $(r_i, m_i) \in \mathcal{R}_i$ in the optimization process. We recall that the later relation means $0 \le r_i \le r_{X_i, m_i}$. In addition, it may be necessary to bound r_i away from zero, in order to show convergence of the scheme. Therefore, we define the closed and convex subset $\mathcal{C} := \Lambda \times \mathcal{R}_{\mathrm{ad}} \subset \Lambda \times \left((\mathcal{U} \times \mathbb{R}^{dI}) \cap \mathcal{R} \right)$ and denote the convex projection onto $\mathcal{C}$ by $\Pi_{\mathcal{C}}$. Since all optimization schemes under consideration to solve

$$\min_{(\lambda, r, m) \in \mathcal{C}} J_{\alpha}(\lambda, r, m)$$

need the gradient of J_{α} as well as the projection operator $\Pi_{\mathcal{C}}$, we provide these quantities in a first step.

5.1.1. Gradient and Projection. The gradient of J_{α} has to satisfy

$$\langle \operatorname{grad} J_{\alpha}(\lambda, r, m), (h_{\lambda}, h_r, h_m) \rangle_{\mathbb{R}^I \times \mathcal{U} \times \mathbb{R}^{dI}} = J'_{\alpha}(\lambda, r, m)(h_{\lambda}, h_r, h_m),$$

where the derivative J'_{α} is known from Theorem 4.2:

$$\langle \operatorname{grad} J_{\alpha}(\lambda, r, m), (h_{\lambda}, h_r, h_m) \rangle_{\mathbb{R}^I \times \mathcal{U} \times \mathbb{R}^{dI}}$$
$$= \langle F(\lambda, r, m) - g, \partial_{\lambda} F(\lambda, r, m) h_{\lambda} + \partial_r F(\lambda, r, m) h_r + \partial_m F(\lambda, r, m) h_m \rangle_{\mathcal{Y}}$$
$$+ \alpha \partial_r \mathrm{Per}(r) h_r$$
$$= \sum_{i=1}^{I} \Big(\langle u|_{\partial X} - g, h_{\lambda, i} v_i|_{\partial X} + u'_{r,i}|_{\partial X} + u'_{m,i}|_{\partial X} \rangle_{\mathcal{Y}}$$
$$+ \alpha \int_{\partial G_i} \mathrm{H}_{\partial G_i} h_{r,i} \cdot \nu \, \mathrm{d}\mu \Big).$$

Herein, $u|_{\partial X} = A \sum_{i=1}^{I} \lambda_i \chi_{G_i}$ and $v_i|_{\partial X} = A \chi_{G_i}$. Moreover, the terms $u'_{r,i}$ and $u_{m,i}$ are the solutions of the transmission boundary value problem (4.10) with h replaced by $h_{r,i}$ and $h_{m,i}$, respectively, as well as Γ replaced by G_i and λ by λ_i.

Obviously, the gradient depends on the choice of the Hilbert space $\mathcal{U}$. We start with the calculation of the L^2 gradient. Later $\mathcal{U}$ will be chosen to be a Sobolev space H^s on the unit sphere, where we can work with an expansion of the parameterization with respect to spherical harmonics. In this context, the H^s gradient is obtained by multiplying the Fourier coefficients associated with spherical harmonics of degree j of the L^2 gradient by $(1 + j^2)^{-s}$ in case $d = 2$ and by $(j + 1/2)^{-2s}$ in case $d = 3$. For more details on Sobolev spaces on the sphere in two and three dimensions see [**Kre89**] and [**FGS98**], respectively.

The components of the L^2 gradient[1] have to satisfy

$$\begin{aligned}
\big(\operatorname{grad} J_\alpha(\lambda, r, m)\big)_{\lambda_i} &= \big\langle F(\lambda, r, m) - g, A\chi_{G_i}\big\rangle_{\mathcal{Y}}, \\
\big(\operatorname{grad} J_\alpha(\lambda, r, m)\big)_{r_i} &= \partial_{r_i} F(\lambda, r, m)^* \big(F(\lambda, r, m) - g\big) \\
&\quad + \alpha \mathrm{H}_{\partial G_i}(\Phi_1 \cdot \nu)\sqrt{\operatorname{gr} \Phi_{r_i}'}, \\
\big(\operatorname{grad} J_\alpha(\lambda, r, m)\big)_{m_i} &= \partial_{m_i} F(\lambda, r, m)^* \big(F(\lambda, r, m) - g\big),
\end{aligned}$$
(5.1)

where Φ_1 is the parameterization of the unit sphere and $\operatorname{gr} \Phi_\rho'$ is the Gramian determinant of the derivative of the parameterization Φ_ρ of $\partial\Gamma$. Since all our numerical experiments in the next section are performed in two dimensions, we specify the components of the gradient in this special case further. We refer to Section 7.1 for a similar treatment in three dimensions.

In case $d = 2$, the second equality of (5.1) reduces to

$$\big(\operatorname{grad} J_\alpha(\lambda, r, m)\big)_{r_i} = \partial_{r_i} F(\lambda, r, m)^* \big(F(\lambda, r, m) - g\big) + \alpha \mathrm{H}_{\partial G_i} r_i. \quad (5.2)$$

Herein, the L^2 adjoint operator of $\partial_{r_i} F(\lambda, r, m)$ is given by

$$\partial_{r_i} F(\lambda, r, m)^* \psi = 2\lambda_i r_i w|_{\partial G_i} \circ \Phi_{r_i} \quad (5.3)$$

with w denoting the solution of the adjoint boundary value problem

$$\begin{aligned}
-\operatorname{div}(D\nabla w) + \sigma_{\mathrm{a}} w &= 0 \quad \text{in } X, \\
2D\frac{\partial w}{\partial \nu} + w &= \psi \quad \text{on } \partial X,
\end{aligned}$$
(5.4)

which has the weak formulation

$$\int_X (D\nabla w \cdot \nabla v + \sigma_{\mathrm{a}} w v)\, \mathrm{d}x + \frac{1}{2}\int_{\partial X} wv\, \mathrm{d}\mu = \frac{1}{2}\int_{\partial X} \psi v\, \mathrm{d}\mu \quad \text{for all } v \in H^1(X).$$

---

[1]We note that we use the subscript λ_i to indicate the ith component in the variable λ of the gradient, that is, $\big\langle (\operatorname{grad} J_\alpha(\lambda, r, m))_{\lambda_i}, h_{\lambda, i}\big\rangle_{\mathcal{Y}} = \partial_{\lambda_i} J_\alpha(\lambda, r, m) h_{\lambda, i}$. This notation is transferred to the variables r and m.

The representation (5.3) of $\partial_{r_i} F(\lambda, r, m)^*$ can be seen from

$$
\begin{aligned}
\langle \partial_{r_i} F(\lambda, r, m) h_{r,i}, \psi \rangle_{\mathcal{Y}} &= \int_{\partial X} u'_{r,i} \psi \, \mathrm{d}\mu \\
&= 2 \int_X (D\nabla w \cdot \nabla u'_{r,i} + \sigma_{\mathrm{a}} w u'_{r,i}) \, \mathrm{d}x + \int_{\partial X} w u'_{r,i} \, \mathrm{d}\mu \\
&= 2\lambda_i \int_{\partial G_i} w \, (h_{r,i} \cdot \nu) \circ \Phi_{r_i}^{-1} \, \mathrm{d}\mu \\
&= \int_{S^1} 2\lambda_i h_{r,i} r_i w \circ \Phi_{r_i} \, \mathrm{d}\mu \\
&= \langle h_{r,i}, \partial_{r_i} F(\lambda, r, m)^* \psi \rangle_{L^2} \,,
\end{aligned}
$$

according to the weak formulation of the transmission boundary value problem (4.9). Similarly, we observe that the adjoint of $\partial_{m_i} F(\lambda, r, m)$, which occurs in the last equation of (5.1), has the form

$$
\partial_{m_i} F(\lambda, r, m)^* \psi = 2\lambda_i \int_{\partial G_i} w\nu \, \mathrm{d}\mu \,. \tag{5.5}
$$

Let us now turn to the derivation of the projection operator onto the set $\mathcal{C}$. It is well-known that the projection in λ onto the interval $\Lambda = \prod [\underline{\lambda}_i, \overline{\lambda}_i]$ is

$$
(\Pi_{\mathcal{C}}^{\lambda} \lambda)_i = \begin{cases} \underline{\lambda}_i \,, & \lambda_i < \underline{\lambda}_i \,, \\ \overline{\lambda}_i \,, & \lambda_i > \overline{\lambda}_i \,, \\ \lambda_i \,, & \text{otherwise} \,. \end{cases}
$$

The projection in (r, m) onto $\mathcal{R}_{\mathrm{ad}}$,

$$
\Pi_{\mathcal{C}}^{(r,m)}(r, m) = \operatorname*{arg\,min}_{(\rho, \xi) \in \mathcal{R}_{\mathrm{ad}}} \| (\rho, \xi) - (r, m) \|_{\mathcal{U} \times \mathbb{R}^{dI}} \,,
$$

depends again on the choice of $\mathcal{U}$ and cannot be expressed explicitly in general. Since in the numerical experiments the iterates stay in $\mathcal{R}_{\mathrm{ad}}$ in case of suitable initial values, the projection onto $\mathcal{R}_{\mathrm{ad}}$ is only of interest from a theoretical point of view.

5.1.2. Projected Gradient Method.
In [HPUU09] the projected gradient method specified in Algorithm 5.1 is presented for constrained optimization in Hilbert spaces.

Algorithm 5.1 Projected Gradient Method

(S0) Choose $(\lambda^0, r^0, m^0) \in \mathcal{C}$.

For $k = 0, 1, 2, \ldots$

(S1) Test for termination.

(S2) Set $(h_\lambda^k, h_r^k, h_m^k) = -\operatorname{grad} J_\alpha(\lambda^k, r^k, m^k)$.

(S3) Choose s_k by a projected step size rule such that

$$J_\alpha\Big(\Pi_{\mathcal{C}}\big((\lambda^k, r^k, m^k) + s_k(h_\lambda^k, h_r^k, h_m^k)\big)\Big) < J_\alpha(\lambda^k, r^k, m^k).$$

(S4) Set $(\lambda^{k+1}, r^{k+1}, m^{k+1}) = \Pi_{\mathcal{C}}\big((\lambda^k, r^k, m^k) + s_k(h_\lambda^k, h_r^k, h_m^k)\big)$.

The step size s_k, occurring in the algorithm, is chosen by the projected Armijo rule: The largest $s_k \in \{\frac{1}{2^n} : n \in \mathbb{N}_0\}$ is chosen such that

$$J_\alpha\Big(\Pi_{\mathcal{C}}\big((\lambda^k, r^k, m^k) + s_k(h_\lambda^k, h_r^k, h_m^k)\big)\Big) - J_\alpha(\lambda^k, r^k, m^k)$$

$$\leq -\frac{\gamma}{s_k}\Big\|\Pi_{\mathcal{C}}\big((\lambda^k, r^k, m^k) + s_k(h_\lambda^k, h_r^k, h_m^k)\big) - (\lambda^k, r^k, m^k)\Big\|^2_{\mathbb{R}^I \times \mathcal{U} \times \mathbb{R}^{dI}}$$

with some constant $\gamma \in \,]0, 1[$.

In [**HPUU09**] a convergence result for the projected gradient method using the projected Armijo rule is established under a Hölder continuity assumption on the gradient of the minimization functional. Though we could only achieve a local Lipschitz continuity of the gradient on $\Lambda \times \mathcal{R}_{\mathrm{ad}}$ with

$$\mathcal{R}_{\mathrm{ad}} = \{(r, m) \in (\mathcal{U} \times \mathbb{R}^{dI}) \cap \mathcal{R} : r_{i,m_i} \geq \varepsilon\}$$

for one $\varepsilon > 0$, we expect Algorithm 5.1 to converge to a critical point also in our setting.

5.1.3. Split Approach. In [**RR07**] Ramlau and Ring propose a split approach, where first the intensity is minimized while freezing the domain and then the domain is updated using the new intensity. Inspired by them, we split the kth iteration into the following two steps:

$$\lambda^{k+1} = \arg\min_{\lambda \in \Lambda} J_\alpha(\lambda, r^k, m^k),$$

$$(r^{k+1}, m^{k+1}) = \Pi_{\mathcal{R}_{\mathrm{ad}}}\big((r^k, m^k) - s_k(h_r^k, h_m^k)\big)$$

with

$$h_r^k = \big(\operatorname{grad} J_\alpha(\lambda^{k+1}, r^k, m^k)\big)_r \quad \text{and} \quad h_m^k = \big(\operatorname{grad} J_\alpha(\lambda^{k+1}, r^k, m^k)\big)_m.$$

The step size s_k is chosen by the projected Armijo rule as above. This leads to Algorithm 5.2.

Algorithm 5.2 Split Approach

(S0) Choose $(\lambda^0, r^0, m^0) \in \mathcal{C}$.

For $k = 0, 1, 2, \ldots$

(S1) Test for termination.

(S2) Calculate $\lambda^{k+1} = \arg\min_{\lambda \in \Lambda} J_\alpha(\lambda, r^k, m^k)$.

(S3) Set $(h_r^k, h_m^k) = -\big(\operatorname{grad} J_\alpha(\lambda^{k+1}, r^k, m^k)\big)_{(r,m)}$.

(S4) Choose s_k by a projected step size rule such that

$$J_\alpha\Big(\lambda^{k+1}, \Pi_{\mathcal{R}_{\mathrm{ad}}}\big((r^k, m^k) + s_k(h_r^k, h_m^k)\big)\Big) < J_\alpha(\lambda^{k+1}, r^k, m^k).$$

(S5) Set $(r^{k+1}, m^{k+1}) = \Pi_{\mathcal{R}_{\mathrm{ad}}}\big((r^k, m^k) + s_k(h_r^k, h_m^k)\big)$.

Let us point out that the optimization problem in step (S2) possesses a solution, since J_α is a quadratic function in λ and the set Λ is compact. Standard quadratic programming can be used to solve this problem [**NW06**]. However, the solution may not be unique unless the matrix $K = \big(\langle A\chi_{G_i}, A\chi_{G_j}\rangle_{L^2}\big)_{i,j}$ is positive definite.

In the case $I = 1$, the optimization problem in (S2) is obviously uniquely solvable. In this situation, similar to the unconstrained case in [**RR07**], the split approach can be viewed as a descent method for the reduced functional

$$\widetilde{J}_\alpha(r, m) = J_\alpha\big(\lambda(r, m), r, m\big) \quad \text{with} \quad \lambda(r, m) = \arg\min_{\lambda \in \Lambda} J_\alpha(\lambda, r, m),$$

as $-\big(\operatorname{grad} J_\alpha(\lambda(r, m), r, m)\big)_{(r,m)}$ is a descent direction for $\widetilde{J}_\alpha(r, m)$ for every (r, m) in the interior of $\mathcal{R}_{\mathrm{ad}}$ such that $\lambda(r, m)$ is in the interior of Λ. This observation is based on the identity

$$\widetilde{J}_\alpha'(r, m) = \partial_\lambda J_\alpha\big(\lambda(r, m), r, m\big)\lambda'(r, m) + \big(\partial_{(r,m)} J_\alpha\big)\big(\lambda(r, m), r, m\big)$$

and the first-order optimality condition

$$\partial_\lambda J_\alpha\big(\lambda(r, m), r, m\big) = 0.$$

5.2. Numerical Experiments

To complete the discussion of the DA-based BLT problem, we present numerical examples of the developed geometric regularization approach. The goals of this section are to see if this technique is feasible to reconstruct photon sources and to understand the still open challenges better. Though all experiments are performed in two dimensions, three-dimensional examples should give similar observations.

5.2.1. Implementation. As mentioned above, we only consider the case $d = 2$ for our experiments. The *PDE Toolbox* of MATLAB is used to compute the solution of the occurring boundary value problems via the Finite Element Method (FEM). More precisely, we use linear elements and the maximal edge size h to be specified later.

For the sake of presentation, we restrict ourselves in this description to the situation where the source term q consists of only one characteristic function: $q = \lambda \chi_G$. Let (r, m) be a parameterization of the searched-for star-shaped domain G. Identifying the unit sphere S^1 with the interval $[0, 2\pi]$, we approximate the function r by a trigonometric polynomial[2] r_M of degree less than M:

$$r(\vartheta) \approx r_M(\vartheta) = \gamma_0 + \sum_{n=1}^{M} \left(\gamma_n^c \cos(n\vartheta) + \gamma_n^s \sin(n\vartheta) \right) \qquad (5.6)$$

for $\vartheta \in [0, 2\pi]$, where

$$\gamma_0 = \frac{1}{2\pi} \int_0^{2\pi} r(\vartheta) \, \mathrm{d}\vartheta \, ,$$

$$\gamma_n^c = \frac{1}{\pi} \int_0^{2\pi} r(\vartheta) \cos(n\vartheta) \, \mathrm{d}\vartheta \, , \qquad (5.7)$$

$$\gamma_n^s = \frac{1}{\pi} \int_0^{2\pi} r(\vartheta) \sin(n\vartheta) \, \mathrm{d}\vartheta \, .$$

Then, all numerical operations are performed on the vector

$$\left(\gamma_0, \gamma_1^c, \ldots, \gamma_M^c, \gamma_1^s, \ldots, \gamma_M^s \right)^\top$$

of coordinates rather than on the function r_M itself.

Our discretization of r requires a matched discretization of the following quantities:

1. the source term q, i.e., the scaled characteristic function $\lambda \chi_G$,
2. the L^2 adjoint of $\partial_r F(\lambda, r, m)$, see (5.3), and
3. the gradient of the perimeter, see (3.5).

Recall that both latter objects appear in the second component of the L^2 gradient $(\operatorname{grad} J_\alpha(\lambda, r, m))_r$ derived in (5.2).

In the following we describe in detail how we handle above quantities:

1. Let G_M be the star-shaped domain parameterized by (r_M, m). Then, we interpolate the scaled characteristic function of G_M in the finite element space to obtain the source function q_h. Now, the FEM solver

---

[2]In three dimensions one can use the expansion into spherical harmonics, see Chapter 7 or [**FGS98**], for instance.

of MATLAB can be straightforwardly applied to evaluate the forward operator A.

2. The L^2 adjoint of $\partial_r F(\lambda, r_M, m)$ is calculated by evaluating the FE solution of the adjoint problem (5.4) at the intersection points of the FE mesh and the boundary of G_M. The resulting piecewise linear function over the boundary of G_M is multiplied by $2\lambda r_M$ and its first $2M + 1$ Fourier coefficients (5.7) are approximated using the trapezoidal rule, where the nodes agree with the intersection points. We emphasize that the quadrature error is of order h, cf. [**HB09**], since the FE solution is in $H^1(\partial G_M)$. Thus, it is of the same order as the error of the FEM, see for instance [**AH05**, Theorem 10.4.1].

3. We calculate the Fourier coefficients (5.7) of the gradient $H_{\partial G_M} r_M$ of the perimeter, i.e., the product of the additive curvature and the parameterization, by the trapezoidal rule, but this time with equidistant nodes. This is possible as $H_{\partial G_M} r_M$ is explicitly known over the interval $[0, 2\pi]$. We choose the number of nodes to be greater than $\max\{2M + 1, 1/h\}$. Thus, the error is at least of order h.

The calculation of the discretized version of the adjoint of $\partial_m F(\lambda, r, m)$, see (5.5), is performed similar to No. 2 above: The FE solution of the adjoint boundary value problem (5.4) is evaluated at the intersection points of the FE mesh and the boundary of G_M. This yields a piecewise linear function, which is multiplied with 2λ times the unit normal ν. The integral of this product over ∂G_M is again approximated by the trapezoidal rule, where the intersection points serve as nodes.

As mentioned in the previous section, we do not implement the projection onto $\mathcal{R}_{\mathrm{ad}}$, since for suitable initial values the iterates stay in this set. Only the projection of λ onto Λ is used.

The Hilbert space $\mathcal{U}$ is chosen to be $H_{\mathrm{p}}^3([0, 2\pi]) \subset C_{\mathrm{p}}^2([0, 2\pi])$, where the subscript p indicates periodic boundary conditions. So the developed theory is applicable. Hettlich [**Het99**] reports only a little difference between numerical simulations in the H^s and in the L^2 setting. Therefore, we also perform some experiments using the L^2 gradient directly.

Three components of the reconstruction process contribute dominantly to the numerical costs: the solutions of the direct and the adjoint boundary value problems (2.29) and (5.4) as well as the determination of the intersection points of the FE mesh and the boundary of G_M, cf. No. 2 above. The direct problem has to be solved repeatedly to determine the step size s_k in both Algorithms 5.1 and 5.2 by the Armijo rule. The other two costly operations are performed only once per iteration step.

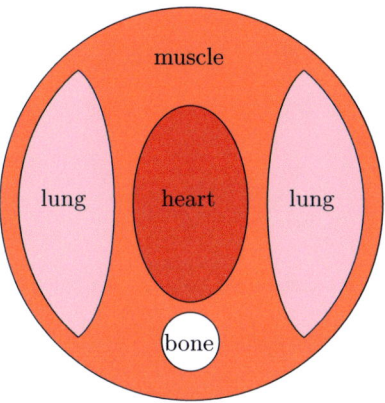

FIGURE 5.1. Sketch of the phantom.

Before we present the used phantom and discuss the numerical experiments, let us explain the termination criterion, which is used in all examples below. Following [**Kel99**, Chapter 5.4.1], the gradient iteration is stopped if

$$\left\|(h_\lambda^k, h_r^k, h_m^k)\right\|_{\mathbb{R}\times\mathcal{U}\times\mathbb{R}^d} \le \tau_a + \tau_r \left\|(h_\lambda^0, h_r^0, h_m^0)\right\|_{\mathbb{R}\times\mathcal{U}\times\mathbb{R}^d}$$

and the split approach if

$$\left\|(h_r^k, h_m^k)\right\|_{\mathbb{R}\times\mathcal{U}} \le \tau_a + \tau_r \left\|(h_r^0, h_m^0)\right\|_{\mathcal{U}\times\mathbb{R}^d},$$

where the notation of Algorithm 5.1 and 5.2 is used. The relative and absolute tolerances are chosen as $\tau_r = \tau_a = 0.005$ for both numerical schemes. Further, the parameter γ in the projected Armijo rule is set to $5 \cdot 10^{-5}$ and the step size s is bounded from below by 2^{-8}.

5.2.2. Phantom. For all our computations in the DA-framework, we use the phantom shown in Figure 5.1, which is also considered in [**Kre08, KR12**] and is approximately the two-dimensional analog of the three-dimensional one presented in [**CWK$^+$05**]. The phantom has the shape of a circular disk with radius 10 and the origin as midpoint. It consists of four different types of tissue, namely bone (B), heart (H), lung (L) and

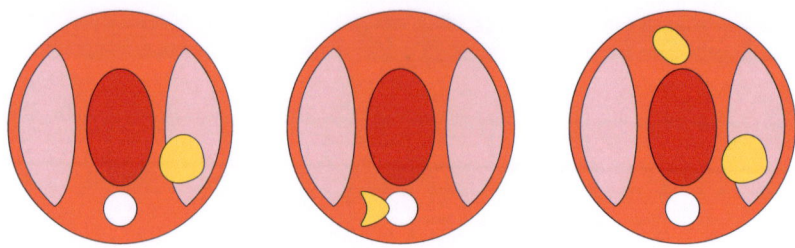

FIGURE 5.2. Sketch of the considered models: Model 1 (left), Model 2 (center), Model 3 (right). The coloring of the phantom is as in Figure 5.1. The yellow region illustrates the bioluminescent source.

muscle (M). They are located in X as follows:

$$B = \left\{ x \in X \colon \sqrt{x_1^2 + (x_2 + 7)^2} \leq 1.5 \right\},$$

$$H = \left\{ x \in X \colon \left(\frac{x_1}{3}\right)^2 + \left(\frac{x_2}{5}\right)^2 \leq 1 \right\},$$

$$L = \left\{ x \in X \colon |x| < 9, \left(\frac{x_1 \pm 6.5}{2.5}\right)^2 + \left(\frac{x_2}{7}\right)^2 < 1 \right\},$$

$$M = X \setminus (B \cup H \cup L).$$

According to [**CWK$^+$05**], realistic optical parameters for these tissues are

$$\sigma_{\mathrm{a}} = \begin{cases} 0.16 & \text{in } B, \\ 0.21 & \text{in } H, \\ 0.22 & \text{in } L, \\ 0.1 & \text{in } M \end{cases} \quad \text{and} \quad \sigma_{\mathrm{s}}' = \begin{cases} 1.28 & \text{in } B, \\ 2.0 & \text{in } H, \\ 2.3 & \text{in } L, \\ 1.2 & \text{in } M. \end{cases}$$

We recall that σ_{s}' is the reduced scattering coefficient and that the diffusion coefficient D is given via

$$D = \frac{1}{3(\sigma_{\mathrm{a}} + \sigma_{\mathrm{s}}')},$$

cf. (2.14).

5.2.3. Model 1. In the first model, the source is placed around the midpoint $(6, -3)$ and its boundary is parameterized by

$$r(\vartheta) = 2 - 0.5 \cos\vartheta + 0.25 \sin\vartheta - 0.1 \sin(3\vartheta),$$

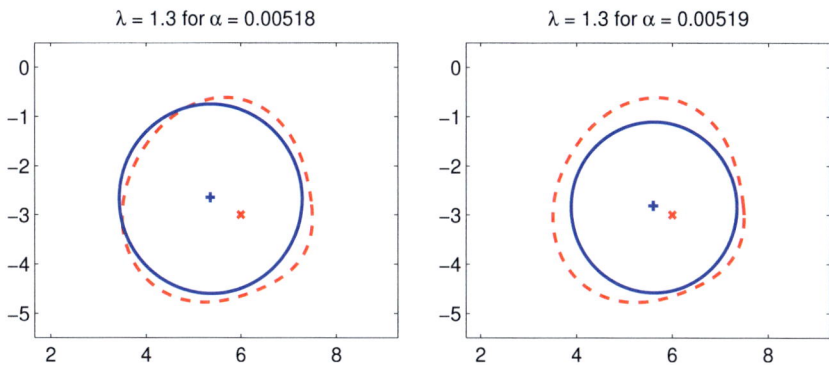

FIGURE 5.3. H^3 setting: Reconstruction (blue solid, midpoint '+') and original source (red dashed, midpoint '×') with $\alpha = 0.00518$ after 201 gradient iterations (left) and with $\alpha = 0.00519$ after 315 gradient iterations (right).

see Figure 5.2 (left) for a sketch of the location in the phantom. The intensity is set to $\lambda = 1$. On a mesh with mesh size 0.2 we produce the synthetic data, whereas the inverse problem is solved on a coarser mesh with $h = 0.5$ in order to avoid the most obvious inverse crime.[3] By linear interpolation we transform the data from the finer grid to the coarser. The relative interpolation error of about 2.7% may be seen as a 'modeling' error.

The maximal degree M of the trigonometric polynomial is set to 8, hence the searched-for parameterization lies in the ansatz space, that is, $r = r_M$ in (5.6). A further discussion on the choice of the maximal degree M is presented in the next paragraph. We choose the regularization parameter α manually by visually inspecting the results. For the intensity λ we allow a variation of 30% of the exact one, i.e., we set $\Lambda = [0.7, 1.3]$. In all experiments based on Model 1 we start with initial values $\lambda^0 = 1.1$, $r^0 \equiv 2.5$ and $m^0 = (5, -2)$.[4]

---

[3]We are aware that we still commit a kind of inverse crime, since we use the diffusion model for generating the data and for solving the inverse problem. In view of the 'modeling' error and the purpose of the numerical experiments, we accept this, though.

[4]In contrast to the numerical experiments in the transport framework in Chapter 7, we do not give the relative discrete L^2 errors of the reconstructions in this chapter. Since all numerical experiments presented in the diffusion framework are performed in two dimensions, the quality of the reconstructions is well assessed by direct inspection.

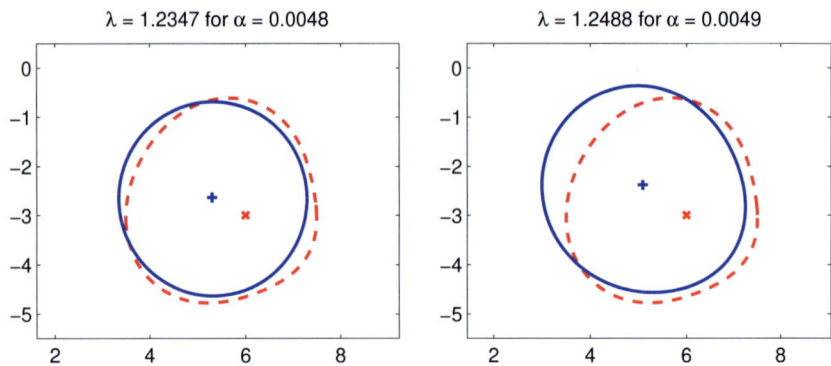

FIGURE 5.4. H^3 vs. L^2 setting: Reconstruction (blue solid, midpoint '+') and original source (red dashed, midpoint '×') in the H^3 setting with $\alpha = 0.0048$ after 265 split approach iterations (left) and in the L^2 setting with $\alpha = 0.0049$ after 148 split approach iterations (right).

5.2.3.1. *Influence of the regularization parameter.* In Figure 5.3 two reconstructions by the gradient method are shown for slightly different regularization parameters. In all our experiments we observe a plateau behavior in the regularization parameter: the reconstruction of (λ, r_M, m) is pretty much stable over a whole range of α-values. However, at certain tipping points the character of the reconstruction changes dramatically. Such a tipping point behavior is demonstrated in Figure 5.3. It originates from the non-uniqueness of the DA-based BLT problem, stated in Lemma 2.10. From the photon density over the boundary we cannot distinguish between a source of small support with high intensity and a low intensity source having large support. It is exactly this kind of non-uniqueness which can be observed in Figure 5.3.

5.2.3.2. *H^3 vs. L^2 setting.* Reconstructions using the split approach in the H^3 and L^2 framework are compared in Figure 5.4. We observe that the L^2 setting leads to a better reconstruction of the shape of the source in the lower right part, which is the side of the domain facing the boundary of X, than in the H^3 regime. In contrast, the shape in the upper left part is not well reconstructed in the L^2 setting, since it is further away from the boundary of X and, consequently, less information arrives in the measurements. In the H^3 setting the reconstructed domain resembles a circular disk due to the intrinsic smoothing property of the H^3 gradient. This characteristic is also observed in the examples given in Figure 5.3.

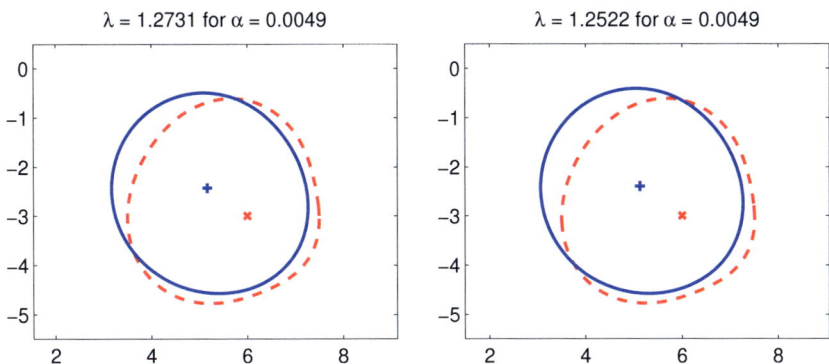

FIGURE 5.5. L^2 setting: Reconstruction (blue solid, midpoint '+') and original source (red dashed, midpoint '×') with $\alpha = 0.0049$ after 163 gradient iterations (left) and with 30% noise level and $\alpha = 0.0049$ after 241 gradient iterations (right).

5.2.3.3. *Noisy data.* In Figure 5.5 (right) we present a numerical experiment where we corrupt the artificial data by 30% relative Gaußian noise with respect to a discrete $L^2(\partial X)$ norm. The difference to the noise-free reconstruction, illustrated in Figure 5.5 (left), is gradual, since the perimeter penalty term as well as the low degree of r_M have a regularizing effect.

So far, we have only discussed the reconstruction of the domain. In all the experiments based on Model 1 we observe that the intensity λ is overestimated. The reason for this is that either the size of the reconstructed source is smaller than the size of the original source or the reconstructed domain is located further away from the boundary. In order to fit the photon density over the surface, this leads in both cases to an overestimation of the intensity.

5.2.4. Model 2. In contrast to the preceding model, the parameterization of the searched-for domain is not explicitly given as an element of the ansatz space in the second model. Inspired from [**Het99**], we consider the kite-shaped source whose boundary is parameterized by

$$x(\vartheta) = \begin{pmatrix} \cos\vartheta + 0.65\big(\cos(2\vartheta) - 1\big) \\ 1.5\sin\vartheta \end{pmatrix} - \begin{pmatrix} 2 \\ 7 \end{pmatrix} \quad \text{for } \vartheta \in [0, 2\pi].$$

An illustration of the location of the source in the phantom is illustrated in Figure 5.2 (center). Though the source is star-shaped with respect to

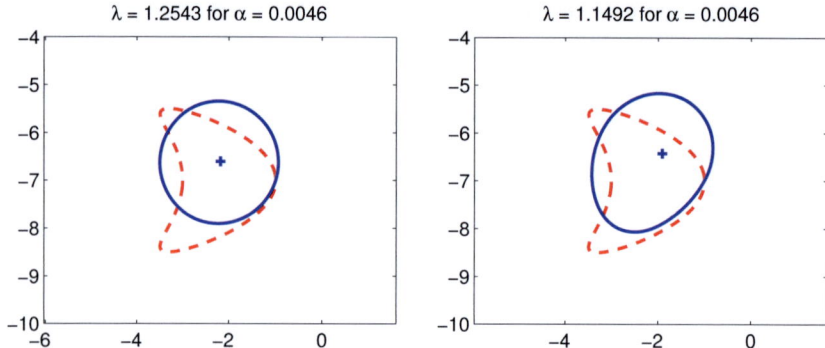

FIGURE 5.6. H^3 vs. L^2 setting: Reconstruction (blue solid, midpoint '+') and original source (red dashed) in the H^3 setting with $\alpha = 0.0046$ after 276 gradient iterations (left) and in the L^2 setting with $\alpha = 0.0046$ after 294 gradient iterations (right).

several points, it is not clear whether there exists a parameterization of the boundary that is a trigonometric polynomial. The intensity of the source is set to $\lambda = 1$. As in Model 1, we generate the synthetic data on a mesh with mesh size 0.2 and solve the inverse problem on a coarser mesh with mesh size $h = 0.5$. This yields a 'modeling' error of 3.6%. To incorporate the *a priori* knowledge on the intensity, we again set $\Lambda = [0.7, 1.3]$. In all experiments of this paragraph the projected gradient method is started with $\lambda^0 = 1.1$.

5.2.4.1. H^3 *vs.* L^2 *setting.* Reconstructions of the kite-shaped source in the H^3 and the L^2 setting are shown in Figure 5.6 (left) and (right), respectively. In both experiments the initial values for the star-shaped domain $m^0 = (-1, -6)$ and $r^0 \equiv 2$ are used. We observe that the H^3 reconstruction is approximately a circular disk centered in the upper half of the kite. In comparison, the L^2 reconstruction is also centered in the upper half but stretches in the direction of the lower tip. The reasons for such a behavior are known from Model 1: The H^3 gradient penalizes higher Fourier coefficients substantially. Due to the non-uniqueness, there exist solutions besides the searched-for domain.

5.2.4.2. *Regularizing effects of α and M.* In the four experiments of Figure 5.7 and Figure 5.8 we focus on the parameterization r of the boundary ∂G and its dependence on the regularization parameter α and the maximal degree M. So, the projected gradient method is initialized with

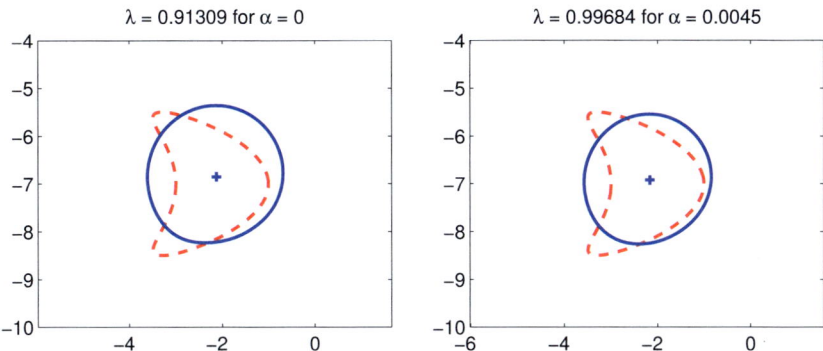

FIGURE 5.7. L^2 setting, $M = 8$: Reconstruction (blue solid, midpoint '+') and original source (red dashed) with $\alpha = 0$ after 24 gradient iterations (left) and with $\alpha = 0.0045$ after 29 gradient iterations (right).

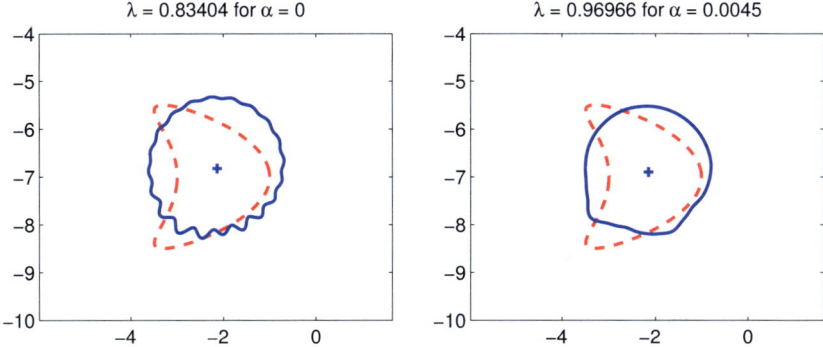

FIGURE 5.8. L^2 setting, $M = 20$: Reconstruction (blue solid, midpoint '+') and original source (red dashed) with $\alpha = 0$ after 54 gradient iterations (left) and with $\alpha = 0.0045$ after 41 gradient iterations (right).

$m^0 = (-2, -7)$ and $r^0 \equiv 1.5$ in all four examples. Only the L^2 setting is used, since we already know the smoothing property of the H^3 gradient.

In Figure 5.7 the unregularized reconstruction (left) is compared with the regularized one (right), where the maximal degree M is set to 8. Though the difference is only slight, we recognize that the size of the regularized source is smaller, since the perimeter is penalized. In both experiments the shape of the kite is not recovered.

For an increased maximal degree, i.e., $M = 20$, the reconstructions are shown in Figure 5.8. Using no regularization by the perimeter term, leads to an oscillating boundary of the reconstruction. These oscillations are effectively damped by the perimeter regularization term.

From the last four experiments we see that not only α but also M serves as regularization parameter in the discretized BLT problem. There are two effects one should keep in mind while choosing M. On the one hand, underestimating M can cause loss of details, since the ansatz space becomes smaller. On the other hand, choosing M too large can produce instability, as seen in Figure 5.8. The numerical costs are, however, marginally influenced by the choice of M.

To finish the discussion of the second model, we note that the kite-shaped source shows us the limitations of the proposed geometric regularization approach. By incorporating the perimeter regularization term, we implicitly assume that the support of the source is rather a circular disk than another more complex geometry, which is reasonable on account of an uniform growth of cell structures. The kite-shaped domain does not really match this assumption and leads to poor reconstructions of the shape. However, even the unregularized reconstruction, see Figure 5.7 (left), resembles more or less a circular disc. This fact shows that the limitation is also a structural one, originating from the non-uniqueness of the DA-based BLT problem.

5.2.5. Model 3. In the third model we consider the situation that two sources are present. The first source is the one known from Model 1, i.e., parameterized by

$$r_1(\vartheta) = 2 - 0.5\cos\vartheta + 0.25\sin\vartheta - 0.1\sin(3\vartheta)$$

with midpoint $m_1 = (6, -3)$ and intensity $\lambda_1 = 1$. A second source with parameterization

$$r_2(\vartheta) = 1.5 - 0.3\sin(2\vartheta)$$

is centered in the point $m_2 = (-1, 7)$ and its intensity set to $\lambda_2 = 0.8$. In Figure 5.2 (right) the location of the two sources in the phantom is illustrated. Once again, artificial data are produced on a finer mesh with mesh size 0.2, whereas a mesh with mesh size $h = 0.5$ is used to solve the inverse problem. This results in a 'modeling' error of 4.6%. In both experiments we set the maximal degree of the trigonometric polynomial to $M = 8$ and the regularization parameter to $\alpha = 0.0032$. Former choice ensures that the searched-for sources are in the ansatz space, i.e., $r = r_M$ in (5.6), without causing instabilities. The latter selection is made by visual inspection of the reconstructions. In addition, the L^2 setting is used.

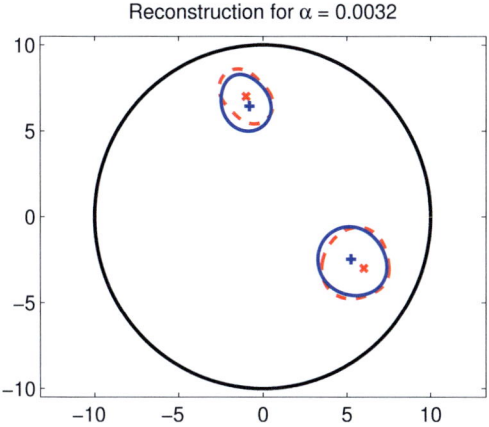

FIGURE 5.9. L^2 setting: Reconstruction (blue solid, midpoint '+') and original source (red dashed, midpoint '×') with $\alpha = 0.0032$ after 343 gradient iterations. The reconstructed intensities are $\lambda_1 = 1.2504$ and $\lambda_2 = 1$.

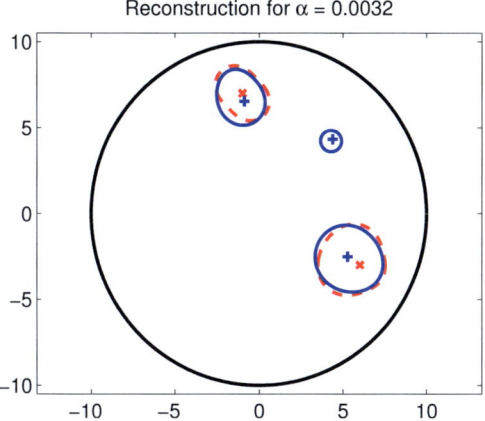

FIGURE 5.10. L^2 setting: Reconstruction (blue solid, midpoint '+') and original source (red dashed, midpoint '×') with $\alpha = 0.0032$ after 345 gradient iterations. The reconstructed intensities are $\lambda_1 = 1.2268$, $\lambda_2 = 0.9997$ and $\lambda_3 = 0.6$.

Figure 5.9 displays a reconstruction given the right number of sources. The projected gradient methods is started with $\lambda_1^0 = 1.1$, $m_1^0 = (5, -2)$, $r_1^0 \equiv 2.5$ and $\lambda_2^0 = 0.9$, $m_2^0 = (0, 6)$, $r_2^0 \equiv 2$. Moreover, we set $\Lambda_1 = [0.7, 1.3]$

and $\Lambda_2 = [0.6, 1]$. Keeping the observations obtained from Model 1 in mind, the support of both sources are rather well reconstructed.

In the experiment whose reconstruction is illustrated in Figure 5.10 the number of sources is overestimated. Three sources are assumed in the solution process of the inverse problems. Besides the two sources known from the previous example, the gradient method is initialized with a third source given by $\lambda_3^0 = 1$, $m_3^0 = (5, 5)$, $r_3^0 \equiv 1.5$. The interval of admissible λ_3-values is set to $\Lambda_3 = [0.6, 1.3]$. We observe that the first two sources are approximately reconstructed as in the previous experiment. The third source moves a little to the inside, its size becomes small and its intensity coincides with the lower bound of the interval Λ_3. We note that the intensity vanishes if 0 is the lower bound of the interval Λ_3.

At this point, let us also remark that the number of sources in the object can roughly be estimated from the measurements. If the sources are not too close to each other and no source is hidden behind another one, the number of local maxima of the photon density on the boundary is a good approximation on the number of sources.

Part III

Radiative Transfer Equation based Bioluminescence Tomography

CHAPTER 6

Domain Derivative of the RTE-based Forward Operator

Let us now turn to the model-specific analysis of the BLT problem in the transport framework. As in Chapter 4 concerning the diffusion model, the key ingredient is the domain derivative of the forward operator. However, the derivation is much more involved. To our knowledge there is no rigorous calculation for a general class of domains. Though we formally calculate the domain derivative about connected domains in Section 6.1, we only can derive it about ball-shaped domains rigorously. Latter is presented in Section 6.2. The reasons why the formal calculation cannot be performed rigorously and why a few other basic approaches cannot be applied is discussed in Section 6.1. We finish this chapter with Section 6.3. There we explain consequences for the minimization problem 2.13, like the one-sided directional derivative of J_α and a further specification of the approximate variational principle, at least for points where the forward operator is domain differentiable.

Before we start with the detailed analysis, we recall the framework of RTE-based BLT set up in Chapter 2. The linear forward operator is defined in (2.25) by

$$A \colon L^1(X) \to L^1\big(\partial_+(X \times \Omega), |\omega \cdot \nu| \, \mathrm{d}\omega \, \mathrm{d}\mu\big) = \mathcal{Y}, \quad q \mapsto u|_{\partial_+(X \times \Omega)}, \quad (6.1)$$

where $u \in W^1_-(X \times \Omega)$ is the solution of the boundary value problem (2.20), that is,

$$\omega \cdot \nabla u(x, \omega) + \sigma_t(x) u(x, \omega) - S u(x, \omega) = q(x), \quad (x, \omega) \in X \times \Omega,$$
$$u(x, \omega) = 0, \quad (x, \omega) \in \partial_-(X \times \Omega), \quad (6.2)$$

with the scattering operator

$$(Su)(x, \omega) = \sigma_s(x) \int_\Omega \eta(x, \omega \cdot \omega') u(x, \omega') \, d\omega'.$$

Taking account of the *a priori* knowledge of piecewise constant sources as in Section 2.3, we obtain the nonlinear forward operator

$$F \colon \Lambda \times \mathcal{L} \to \mathcal{Y}, \quad (\lambda, G) \mapsto \sum_{i=1}^{I} \lambda_i A \chi_{G_i}, \quad (6.3)$$

compare (2.35).

6.1. Formal Calculation and Discussion

As mentioned above, we formally derive the domain derivative of F in this section. This derivation is followed by an argument why this cannot be performed rigorously and why also other rigorous approaches fail. These observations lead then to the technical but rigorous calculation of the domain derivative about a ball in the upcoming section 6.2.

For the sake of simplicity, we assume in the subsequent presentation that there is only one source, i.e., $I = 1$.

6.1.1. Formal Calculation of the Domain Derivative of F. For the formal derivative of F with respect to the geometric variable, we decompose the operator $F(\lambda, \cdot)$ as in Section 4.1.1:

$$F(\lambda, G) = A \circ Q(G)$$

with the map

$$Q \colon G \mapsto \lambda \chi_G.$$

We ignore the domains and the image spaces of these functions as well as smoothness assumptions due to the formal nature of the calculation. Following the calculations in Section 4.1.1, the domain derivative of Q about Γ in direction h is given by

$$Q'(\Gamma) h = \lambda h_\nu \delta_{\partial \Gamma},$$

cf. (4.8). We apply the linear forward operator A, defined in (6.1), to this equation and obtain the formal domain derivative of the nonlinear forward operator $F(\lambda, \cdot)$, specified in (6.3), about Γ in direction h

$$\partial_\Gamma F(\lambda, \Gamma) h = \lambda A(h_\nu \delta_{\partial \Gamma}). \quad (6.4)$$

6.1.2. Discussion of the Formal and Other Approaches. [1]

Though we found in the last paragraph a formal way to calculate the domain derivative of the forward operator, we doubt that this derivation can be performed rigorously. To differentiate Q rigorously, we need a continuous trace operator on the space of test functions, compare the calculations in Section 4.1.1. Since functions in $W^{1,1}(X)$ have a trace in $L^1(\partial\Gamma)$ [**AF03**], the operator Q is differentiable as a mapping from the set of smooth domains $\mathcal{S}$ to the dual space $W^{-1,\infty}(X)$ of $W^{1,1}(X)$. Thus, the forward operator F would be domain differentiable if the operator A defined in (6.1) was bounded from $W^{-1,\infty}(X)$ to $\mathcal{Y}$.[2] We are not aware of any statement proving or disproving this continuity. However, we think that it does not hold in general. The reason lies in the fact that the solution of the transport equation (6.2) is marginally smoother in the spatial variable than the source term: Only the directional derivatives of the solution are bounded in the same norm as the source function, but not the derivative itself.

Nevertheless, the calculation of the previous subsection can be rigorously performed in the following setting: in two dimensions, no scattering happens, and the mapping properties of A are relaxed. This is the framework of SPECT. To our knowledge, the domain derivative of the SPECT forward operator has not been derived before. As it is an interesting result on its own, we present it in an excursus in Appendix E.

In Section 4.1.2 we mentioned and referred to another technique for the derivation of the domain derivative of the DA-based BLT forward operator about general C^2 shapes. In this approach one applies a change of variables to the weak formulation of the boundary value problem with perturbed quantities and then estimates the difference between the weak formulations cleverly. In [**Het99**] this method is used for the calculation of the domain derivative for a broad class of inverse problems involving second-order elliptic differential equations. By contrast, this approach seems not to work for the BLT forward operator based on the radiative transfer equation.

---

[1]In this subsection we discuss why the technique above and other standard approaches are not applicable to derive the domain derivative in RTE-based BLT rigorously. This serves to motivate the rather ugly calculations in the next section, but is not essential to understand the following presentation. So, it might be skipped by the reader.

[2]If the searched-for domain Γ is contained in $X_0 \subset \overline{X_0} \subset X$, it is sufficient to have continuity for sources supported in X_0 only.

In order to describe the occurring difficulties, we recall and introduce some notations: Let $\Gamma \in \mathcal{S}$ be a smooth domain and $\Gamma_h = \varphi(\Gamma)$ its perturbed version, where $\varphi = \mathrm{id} + h$ and $h \in C_0^1(X, \mathbb{R}^d)$. The Jacobian matrix of the function φ is denoted by $\mathcal{J}_\varphi$. Furthermore, let u and u_h be the solutions of the boundary value problem (6.2) with source term $\lambda \chi_\Gamma$ and $\lambda \chi_{\Gamma_h}$, respectively. The crucial point in this approach is to estimate the difference of the original and perturbed solution in a weak formulation of the radiative transfer equation. Weak formulations can be found in [**Ago98, ES12**], which are only stated in a Hilbert space setting though. The weak characterizations involve the derivative of the solution or of the test function in direction ω. However, instead of comparing u and u_h directly, the difference of u and $\widetilde{u}_h = u_h \circ \varphi$ is considered in order to have matching jump interfaces. This leads to the problem that, after a change of variables, terms like $(\mathcal{J}_\varphi^{-1}(x)\omega)^T \nabla \widetilde{u}_h(x, \omega)$ arise. It is open if the derivatives in these directions exist, since only existence of the directional derivatives $\omega^T \nabla \widetilde{u}_h(x, \omega)$ is ensured for solutions of the transport equation. Consequently, this approach can be a applied for a formal derivation. Due to the open smoothness question, it is not clear if it is suited for a rigorous calculation.

In the literature, standard results on boundary and domain integrals, given e.g. in [**DZ11**], are often used to differentiate a shape dependent functional with respect to the shape. To apply the basic formulas, the domain of integration has to be the shape or the boundary of the shape with respect to which one differentiates. This technique is employed in [**KRR11**], for instance, to differentiate an L^2 residual functional for the two-dimensional attenuated Radon transform. For the sake of completeness, we note that the norm term in the functional J_α does not obey the required form for this approach when scattering is present.

To complete this discussion, we point out the following result, which we will obtain in the next section: Let us consider the Hilbert space framework, i.e., the L^2 setting. Then, we see in Remark 6.7 that the solution u' of the boundary value problem (6.2) with source term $\lambda h_\nu \delta_{\partial G}$ is not an element in $L^2(X \times \Omega)$ when G is a ball and no scattering occurs. Even for every neighborhood U of ∂X the L^2 norm of $u' \chi_U$ is unbounded. Thus, a rigorous derivation of the domain derivative of F in the L^p setting with $p \geq 2$ is not possible.

6.2. Rigorous Derivation of the Domain Derivative of F about a Ball

Since we observed in the discussion above that the standard (and elegant) approaches do not work out, we rigorously calculate the domain derivative in this section in a brute force manner. This derivation holds only for ball-shaped sources so far. However, it might be extended to more general shapes, like convex domains diffeomorphic to the ball, tracing this case back to the ball-shaped one.

So, let us assume in this section that $\Gamma \subset X$ is a ball of radius R centered w.l.o.g. in the origin, i.e., $\Gamma = B_R(0)$. Additionally, let $\partial\Gamma \cap \partial X = \emptyset$, which means that Γ is bounded away from the boundary of X. As we consider only one source, we set $I = 1$ in the subsequent analysis.

Before we start to calculate the domain derivative of F about Γ, we recall a few notations and results from Section 2.2.1 and Section 3.2.1: For the differential operator on the left-hand side of the radiative transfer equation (6.2) we introduce the mapping

$$L\colon \mathcal{D}(L) \subset L^1(X \times \Omega) \to L^1(X \times \Omega)\,, \quad u \mapsto Lu = (\omega \cdot \nabla + \sigma_{\mathrm{t}} I - S)u$$

with $\mathcal{D}(L) = W_-^1(X \times \Omega)$. From Corollary 2.5 we know that the operator L^{-1} is bounded from $L^1(X \times \Omega)$ into itself. In equation (2.24) we recast the radiative transfer equation (6.2) as integral equation

$$(I - \mathcal{K})u = \mathcal{P}q\,,$$

where the integral operators $\mathcal{K}$ and $\mathcal{P}$ are defined by

$$\mathcal{K}v(x,\omega) = \int_0^{\tau_-(x,\omega)} \exp\left(-\int_0^t \sigma_{\mathrm{t}}(x - s\omega)\,\mathrm{d}s\right) Sv(x - t\omega, \omega)\,\mathrm{d}t\,,$$

$$\mathcal{P}v(x,\omega) = \int_0^{\tau_-(x,\omega)} \exp\left(-\int_0^t \sigma_{\mathrm{t}}(x - s\omega)\,\mathrm{d}s\right) v(x - t\omega, \omega)\,\mathrm{d}t$$

for $(x, \omega) \in X \times \Omega$. Herein, $\tau_-(x,\omega)$ is the time of travel given by

$$\tau_-(x,\omega) = \sup\{t\colon x - s\omega \in X \text{ for } 0 \le s < t\}\,.$$

Furthermore, for a vector field $h \in C_0^1(X, \mathbb{R}^d)$ we denote by Γ_h the perturbed domain

$$\Gamma_h = \{x + h(x)\colon x \in \Gamma\}\,.$$

The subscript h is also used for other quantities to indicate that Γ is substituted by Γ_h.

Our aim is to differentiate $F(\lambda, \cdot)$ about Γ, that is, we want to find an operator $\partial_\Gamma F(\lambda, \Gamma) \in \mathcal{L}(C_0^1, \mathcal{Y})$ such that

$$\|F(\lambda, \Gamma_h) - F(\lambda, \Gamma) - \partial_\Gamma F(\lambda, \Gamma)h\|_{\mathcal{Y}} = o\big(\|h\|_{C^1}\big).$$

Since in [**Hyv07**, Lemma 3.4] it is shown that for smooth domains G it is sufficient to consider perturbations in normal direction to derive the domain derivative, we will only take perturbations of the form $h = h_\nu \nu$ with $h_\nu = h \cdot \nu$ into account in the following analysis. Then, the asymptotic behavior in the characterization of the domain derivative reads

$$\|F(\lambda, \Gamma_h) - F(\lambda, \Gamma) - \partial_\Gamma F(\lambda, \Gamma)h\|_{\mathcal{Y}} = o\big(\|h_\nu\|_{C^1}\big).$$

In our derivation we proceed as follows: At first, we decompose F as

$$F(\lambda, G) = \lambda\gamma_+(I - \mathcal{K})^{-1}\widetilde{F}(G) \quad \text{with} \quad \widetilde{F}(G) = \mathcal{P}\chi_G \qquad (6.5)$$

and then calculate the pointwise domain derivative of $\widetilde{F}$ about Γ, i.e., the operator $\widetilde{F}'(\Gamma)$ such that

$$|\widetilde{F}(\Gamma_h)(x,\omega) - \widetilde{F}(\Gamma)(x,\omega) - \big(\widetilde{F}'(\Gamma)h\big)(x,\omega)| = o\big(\|h_\nu\|_{C^1}\big)$$

for almost all $(x,\omega) \in X \times \Omega$. In the next step we show that this estimate not only holds pointwise, but in $L^1(X \times \Omega)$. So $\widetilde{F}'(\Gamma)$ is also the regular domain derivative. In the last step we verify that the trace of $(I - \mathcal{K})^{-1}\widetilde{F}'(\Gamma)h$ exists in $\mathcal{Y}$ and thus $\lambda\gamma_+(I - \mathcal{K})^{-1}\widetilde{F}'(\Gamma)$ is the domain derivative of $F(\lambda, \cdot)$ about Γ.

6.2.1. Preliminaries. In the decomposition (6.5) the inverse of $I - \mathcal{K}$ appears, whose existence we have not discussed yet. This question is addressed in different spaces in the literature [**Bal09, CS99, SU08**]. We only restate the results from [**CS99**, Proposition 2.4], as it is the setting we work in here.

Lemma 6.1. *Let the subcritical condition* (2.18) *hold. Then, the operators* $\mathcal{K}$ *and* $\mathcal{P}$ *are bounded from* $L^1(X \times \Omega)$ *into itself and* $\mathcal{K} = \mathcal{P}S$ *holds. Moreover,* $I - \mathcal{K}$ *is invertible in* $L^1(X \times \Omega)$ *with*

$$(I - \mathcal{K})^{-1} = I + L^{-1}S. \qquad (6.6)$$

The identity (6.6) plays an important role in the last step of the calculation of the domain derivative of F, where we carry over the differentiability from $\widetilde{F}$ to $F(\lambda, \cdot)$.

In order to simplify the notation, we introduce the abbreviation E_{σ_t} for the attenuation term in the integral operators $\mathcal{P}$ and $\mathcal{K}$, that is,

$$E_{\sigma_t}(x,\omega,t) = \exp\left(-\int_0^t \sigma_t(x - s\omega)\,\mathrm{d}s\right) \qquad (6.7)$$

for $(x, \omega, t) \in X \times \Omega \times \mathbb{R}$. The operators $\mathcal{K}$ and $\mathcal{P}$ now read

$$\mathcal{K}v(x, \omega) = \int_0^{\tau_-(x,\omega)} E_{\sigma_t}(x, \omega, t) Sv(x - t\omega, \omega) \, dt \,,$$

$$\mathcal{P}v(x, \omega) = \int_0^{\tau_-(x,\omega)} E_{\sigma_t}(x, \omega, t) v(x - t\omega, \omega) \, dt \,.$$

Moreover, we often have to consider the intersection of the line segment

$$l_{x,\omega} = \{x - t\omega \colon t \in [0, \tau_-(x, \omega)]\}$$

with the ball $\Gamma = B_R(0)$ and the intersection of $l_{x,\omega}$ with the perturbed domain Γ_h in the subsequent analysis of the operators $\widetilde{F}$ and F. To simplify the presentation later, we introduce the notation and some important geometric properties in this paragraph.

6.2.1.1. *Intersection points.* Let $(x, \omega) \in X \times \Omega$. We can write

$$x = x^T \omega \omega + x^T \omega_\perp \omega_\perp \,,$$

where we choose $\omega_\perp \in \Omega$ such that $\omega \cdot \omega_\perp = 0$ and, in addition, $x \cdot (\omega \times \omega_\perp) = 0$ if $d = 3$. To distinguish whether $l_{x,\omega}$ intersects Γ or not, we define the visibility function

$$\psi(x, \omega) = \begin{cases} 1 \,, & l_{x,\omega} \cap \Gamma \neq \emptyset \,, \\ 0 \,, & \text{otherwise} \,. \end{cases} \tag{6.8}$$

With the vector $\omega_\perp$ defined as above we obtain for $x \notin \overline{\Gamma}$ the equivalence

$$\psi(x, \omega) = 1 \iff x^T \omega > 0 \text{ and } x^T \omega_\perp \in \,]-R, R[\,. \tag{6.9}$$

For $(x, \omega) \in X \times \Omega$ with $\psi(x, \omega) = 1$ the intersection points of the line $\{x - t\omega \colon t \in \mathbb{R}\}$ and $\partial\Gamma$ are given by

$$p_i = p_i(x, \omega) = x^T \omega_\perp \omega_\perp + (-1)^i \sqrt{R^2 - (x^T \omega_\perp)^2} \, \omega = x - \tau_i \omega \tag{6.10}$$

with

$$\tau_i = \tau_i(x, \omega) = x^T \omega - (-1)^i \sqrt{R^2 - (x^T \omega_\perp)^2} \quad \text{and} \quad i = 1, 2 \,, \tag{6.11}$$

see also Figure 6.1. Notice that we consider here the whole line to handle the case $x \in \Gamma$ and $x \in X \setminus \overline{\Gamma}$ combined.

For a perturbation $h = h_\nu \nu$ of Γ we introduce the corresponding quantities. Let

$$\psi_h(x, \omega) = \begin{cases} 1 \,, & l_{x,\omega} \cap \Gamma_h \neq \emptyset \,, \\ 0 \,, & \text{otherwise} \,, \end{cases} \tag{6.12}$$

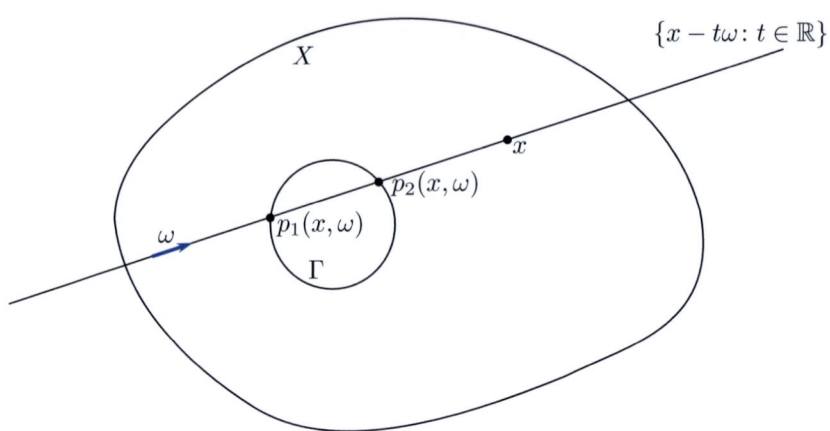

FIGURE 6.1. Sketch of the intersection points of the line $\{x - t\omega : t \in \mathbb{R}\}$ with Γ.

be the visibility function. Given that $\psi_h(x, \omega) = 1$, the line $\{x - t\omega : t \in \mathbb{R}\}$ intersects $\partial\Gamma_h$ in the points

$$p_i^h = p_i^h(x, \omega) = x - \tau_i^h \omega$$

with

$$\tau_i^h = \tau_i^h(x, \omega) = \tau_i - \Delta\tau_i = \tau_i(x, \omega) - \Delta\tau_i(x, \omega) \quad \text{and} \quad i = 1, 2 \,.$$

The difference $\Delta\tau_i$ between τ_i^h and τ_i depends on h. The term is investigated in the following paragraph.

Later we also use the notations $\tau_i(x, \omega)$ and $\tau_i^h(x, \omega)$ for points $(x, \omega) \in X \times \Omega$ that do not satisfy $\psi(x, \omega) = 1$ and $\psi_h(x, \omega) = 1$, respectively. In such situations we set $\tau_i(x, \omega) = \infty$ and $\tau_i^h(x, \omega) = \infty$, respectively.

6.2.1.2. *Asymptotics of* $|\Delta\tau_i|$. An important role in the subsequent calculations plays the asymptotic behavior of $\Delta\tau_i$ for $h \to 0$ as well as an upper bound. We will derive both here.

As the results are local at the intersection point p_i on the boundary $\partial\Gamma$, it is sufficient to consider the planar case in the proofs. The three-dimensional result follows by examination of the planes spanned by the vectors $\nu(p_i)$ and ω.

Lemma 6.2 (Estimate of $\Delta\tau_i$). *For* $(x, \omega) \in X \times \Omega$ *with* $\psi(x, \omega) = \psi_h(x, \omega) = 1$ *holds*

$$|\Delta\tau_i(x, \omega)| \le 3 \frac{\|h_\nu\|_\infty}{|\omega \cdot \nu(p_i(x, \omega))|} \,.$$

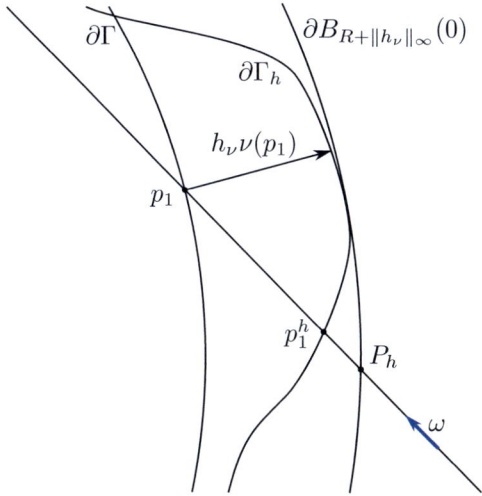

FIGURE 6.2. Sketch of the geometry in the proof of Lemma 6.2.

PROOF. For the sake of presentation, we omit the dependence of p_i and $\Delta\tau_i$ on (x,ω) in this proof. Moreover, we show the statement only for $i = 1$. The bounds for $i = 2$ can be derived in a similar way. To prove the assertion for $i = 1$, we distinguish between the cases $h_\nu(p_1) \geq 0$ and $h_\nu(p_1) < 0$. W.l.o.g. we consider the case $d = 2$.

Let us start with the first case, i.e., $h_\nu(p_1) \geq 0$. As p_1 is on the incoming boundary of $\Gamma = B_R(0)$, the inequality $\omega \cdot \nu(p_1) < 0$ and the identity $|p_1| = R$ hold. We set P_h as intersection point of $l_{p_1,\omega}$ and $\partial B_{R+\|h_\nu\|_\infty}(0)$, that is,

$$P_h = p_1 - \gamma\omega \quad \text{with } \gamma \geq 0\,.$$

In Figure 6.2 the geometry is sketched. Obviously, $\gamma \geq \Delta\tau_1 \geq 0$. Multiplying P_h by $\nu(p_1)$, we obtain

$$R + \gamma|\omega \cdot \nu(p_1)| = (p_1 - \gamma\omega) \cdot \nu(p_1) = P_h \cdot \nu(p_1)$$
$$= (R + \|h_\nu\|_\infty)\frac{P_h}{|P_h|} \cdot \nu(p_1) \leq R + \|h_\nu\|_\infty\,.$$

Therefore,

$$|\Delta\tau_1| \leq \gamma \leq \frac{\|h_\nu\|_\infty}{|\omega \cdot \nu(p_1)|}\,.$$

The case $h_\nu(p_1) < 0$ is a little more involved. Again we have $\omega \cdot \nu(p_1) < 0$ and $|p_1| = R$. Let P_h be the intersection point of $\{x - t\omega \colon t \in \mathbb{R}\}$ and

$\partial B_{R-\|h_\nu\|_\infty}(0)$ such that

$$P_h = p_1 - \gamma\omega \quad \text{and} \quad \frac{P_h}{|P_h|} \cdot \omega \leq 0.$$

It is easy to see that $\gamma \leq \Delta\tau_1 \leq 0$. Furthermore, we observe that

$$R - \|h_\nu\|_\infty = P_h \cdot \frac{P_h}{|P_h|} = (p_1 - \gamma\omega) \cdot \frac{P_h}{|P_h|}$$

$$= R\nu(p_1) \cdot \frac{P_h}{|P_h|} - |\gamma| \left| \omega \cdot \frac{P_h}{|P_h|} \right| \leq R - |\gamma| \left| \omega \cdot \frac{P_h}{|P_h|} \right|,$$

which is equivalent to

$$\|h_\nu\|_\infty \geq |\gamma| \left| \omega \cdot \frac{P_h}{|P_h|} \right|.$$

The last term on the right-hand side can be rewritten as

$$\left| \omega \cdot \frac{P_h}{|P_h|} \right| = -\omega \cdot \frac{P_h}{|P_h|} = -\frac{1}{R - \|h_\nu\|_\infty}(p_1 - \gamma\omega) \cdot \omega$$

$$= \frac{1}{R - \|h_\nu\|_\infty} \left(R|\omega \cdot \nu(p_1)| - |\gamma| \right).$$

Consequently,

$$\|h_\nu\|_\infty \geq \frac{|\gamma|}{R - \|h_\nu\|_\infty} \left(R|\omega \cdot \nu(p_1)| - |\gamma| \right). \tag{6.13}$$

By the nature of γ it is clear that $|\gamma|$ is bounded from above by half the length of the chord of $\partial B_R(0)$ that is tangential to $\partial B_{R-\|h_\nu\|_\infty}(0)$. Thus,

$$|\gamma| \leq \sqrt{2\|h_\nu\|_\infty R - \|h_\nu\|_\infty^2}.$$

Using this in (6.13) implies

$$|\gamma||\omega \cdot \nu(p_1)| \leq \frac{R - \|h_\nu\|_\infty}{R}\|h_\nu\|_\infty + \frac{|\gamma|^2}{R}$$

$$\leq \|h_\nu\|_\infty + \frac{2\|h_\nu\|_\infty R - \|h_\nu\|_\infty^2}{R}$$

$$\leq 3\|h_\nu\|_\infty.$$

We finally obtain

$$|\Delta\tau_1| \leq |\gamma| \leq 3\frac{\|h_\nu\|_\infty}{|\omega \cdot \nu(p_1)|}.$$

$\square$

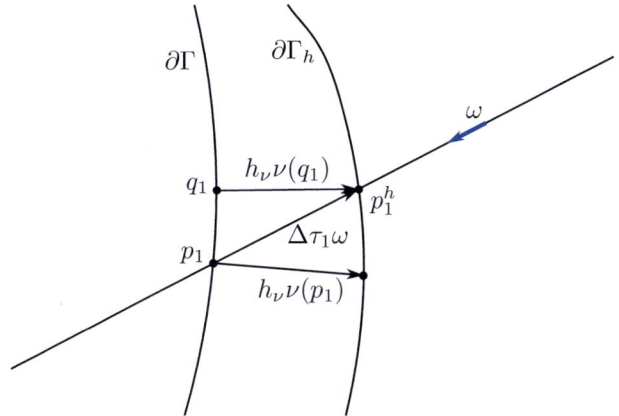

FIGURE 6.3. Sketch of the geometry in the proof of Lemma 6.3 for $i = 1$.

Lemma 6.3 (Asymptotic behavior of $\Delta \tau_i$). *Let* $(x, \omega) \in X \times \Omega$ *with* $\psi(x, \omega) = \psi_h(x, \omega) = 1$. *Then, we have*

$$\Delta \tau_i(x, \omega) = \frac{h_\nu\big(p_i(x, \omega)\big)}{\omega \cdot \nu\big(p_i(x, \omega)\big)} + o\big(\|h_\nu\|_{C^1}\big) \quad as \ h \to 0.$$

PROOF. For the sake of presentation, we omit the dependence of p_i and $\Delta \tau_i$ on (x, ω) in this proof. W.l.o.g. we consider the case $d = 2$.

The point p_i^h can be written as $p_i + \Delta \tau_i \omega$ and in the form $q_i + h_\nu \nu(q_i)$ for a suitable $q_i \in \partial \Gamma$, see Figure 6.3 for a sketch. As $p_i, q_i \in \partial \Gamma = \partial B_R(0)$, there exist $\phi \in [0, 2\pi[$ and $s \in \,]-\pi, \pi]$ with

$$p_i = R \begin{pmatrix} \cos \phi \\ \sin \phi \end{pmatrix} \quad and \quad q_i = R \begin{pmatrix} \cos(\phi + s) \\ \sin(\phi + s) \end{pmatrix}.$$

Multiplying the identity $p_i + \Delta \tau_i \omega = q_i + h_\nu \nu(q_i)$ by the normal vector $\nu(p_i) = (\cos \phi, \sin \phi)^T$, we obtain

$$R + \Delta \tau_i \nu(p_i)^T \omega = \big(R + h_\nu(q_i)\big) \cos s.$$

A Taylor expansion of the cosine yields

$$\Delta \tau_i = \frac{h_\nu(q_i)}{\omega \cdot \nu(p_i)} + O(|s|^2). \tag{6.14}$$

Furthermore, the multiplication of the identity $p_i + \Delta \tau_i \omega = q_i + h_\nu \nu(q_i)$ with the tangential vector $\nu_\perp(p_i) = \nu(p_i)_\perp = (-\sin \phi, \cos \phi)^T$ leads to

$$\Delta \tau_i \nu_\perp(p_i)^T \omega = \big(R + h_\nu(q_i)\big) \sin s,$$

which can be reformulated as

$$s = \arcsin\left(\frac{\Delta\tau_i \nu_\perp(p_i)^T \omega}{R + h_\nu(q_i)}\right) = \frac{\nu_\perp(p_i) \cdot \omega}{R + h_\nu(q_i)}\Delta\tau_i + O(|\Delta\tau_i|^2)\,.$$

Since the estimate

$$|\Delta\tau_i| \le \frac{3\|h_\nu\|_\infty}{|\omega \cdot \nu(p_i)|}$$

holds according to Lemma 6.2, it follows that s is proportional to $\|h_\nu\|_\infty$ up to higher order terms.

Applying the mean value theorem to the function $s \mapsto h_\nu(q_i(s))$, we observe

$$h_\nu(q_i) = h_\nu(p_i) + h'_\nu(\widetilde{q}_i)\widetilde{q}'_i s + O(|s|^2)\,,$$

where

$$\widetilde{q}_i = R\begin{pmatrix}\cos(\phi+\widetilde{s})\\\sin(\phi+\widetilde{s})\end{pmatrix}, \quad \widetilde{q}'_i = R\begin{pmatrix}-\sin(\phi+\widetilde{s})\\\cos(\phi+\widetilde{s})\end{pmatrix} \quad \text{and} \quad \widetilde{s} \in\,]0,s[\,.$$

Combining this with (6.14) and the proportionality of s and $\|h_\nu\|_\infty$, we conclude that

$$\Delta\tau_i = \frac{h_\nu(p_i)}{\omega \cdot \nu(p_i)} + o\big(\|h_\nu\|_{C^1}\big)\,.$$

$\square$

6.2.2. Pointwise Domain Derivative of $\widetilde{F}$.

After the preparations in the previous section, we begin with the differentiation of F by calculating the pointwise domain derivative of $\widetilde{F}$. In other words, we want to find a function $H(x,\omega)$ depending linearly on $h = h_\nu\nu$ such that

$$|f_h(x,\omega) - f(x,\omega) - H(x,\omega)| = o\big(\|h_\nu\|_{C^1}\big)$$

for almost all $(x,\omega) \in X \times \Omega$, where $f = \mathcal{P}\chi_\Gamma$ and $f_h = \mathcal{P}\chi_{\Gamma_h}$.

Let us specify the latter two functions. For $(x,\omega) \in X \times \Omega$ we observe

$$f(x,\omega) = \widetilde{F}(\Gamma)(x,\omega) = (\mathcal{P}\chi_\Gamma)(x,\omega)$$

$$= \psi(x,\omega)\int_0^{\tau_-(x,\omega)} E_{\sigma_t}(x,\omega,t)\chi_\Gamma(x - t\omega)\,\mathrm{d}t$$

$$= \psi(x,\omega)\int_0^{\tau_-(x,\omega)} E_{\sigma_t}(x,\omega,t)\chi_{B_R(0)}\big(x^T\omega_\perp\omega_\perp + (x^T\omega - t)\omega\big)\,\mathrm{d}t$$

$$= \psi(x,\omega)\int_0^{\tau_-(x,\omega)} E_{\sigma_t}(x,\omega,t)\chi_{[\tau_2(x,\omega),\tau_1(x,\omega)]}(t)\,\mathrm{d}t$$

$$= \psi(x,\omega)\int_{\max\{0,\tau_2(x,\omega)\}}^{\tau_1(x,\omega)} E_{\sigma_t}(x,\omega,t)\,\mathrm{d}t \qquad\qquad (6.15)$$

and, analogously, for the perturbed version

$$f_h(x,\omega) = \widetilde{F}(\Gamma_h)(x,\omega) = (\mathcal{P}\chi_{\Gamma_h})(x,\omega)$$
$$= \psi_h(x,\omega) \int_{\max\{0,\tau_2(x,\omega)-\Delta\tau_2(x,\omega)\}}^{\tau_1(x,\omega)-\Delta\tau_1(x,\omega)} E_{\sigma_t}(x,\omega,t)\,\mathrm{d}t\,. \tag{6.16}$$

We recall that the attenuation function E_{σ_t}, the visibility function ψ and its perturbed variant ψ_h are defined in (6.7), (6.8) and (6.12), respectively.

The form of f_h and f together with Lemma 6.3 motivates the guess[3]

$$H(x,\omega) \tag{6.17}$$
$$= \int_0^{\tau_-(x,\omega)} E_{\sigma_t}(x,\omega,t)\frac{h_\nu(x-t\omega)}{\omega\cdot\nu(x-t\omega)}\Big(\delta\big(t-\tau_2(x,\omega)\big) - \delta\big(t-\tau_1(x,\omega)\big)\Big)\,\mathrm{d}t\,.$$

Herein, δ denotes the one-dimensional delta distribution. This is indeed the pointwise domain derivative, as we see in the next theorem.

Theorem 6.4. *For almost all $(x,\omega) \in X \times \Omega$ holds*

$$\frac{1}{\|h_\nu\|_{C^1}}\big|f_h(x,\omega) - f(x,\omega) - H(x,\omega)\big| \to 0 \quad \text{as } h \to 0\,.$$

PROOF. To show the statement, we consider all possible combinations of values of $\psi(x,\omega)$ and $\chi_\Gamma(x)$ separately. For the sake of presentation, we omit the dependency of p_i, τ_i and $\Delta\tau_i$ on (x,ω).

Case $\psi(x,\omega) = 1$ and $x \notin \overline{\Gamma}$:
Then, $\psi_h(x,\omega) = 1$ and $x \notin \overline{\Gamma_h}$ for sufficiently small h. Under these conditions we have

$$f_h(x,\omega) - f(x,\omega) = \int_{\tau_2-\Delta\tau_2}^{\tau_2} E_{\sigma_t}(x,\omega,t)\,\mathrm{d}t + \int_{\tau_1}^{\tau_1-\Delta\tau_1} E_{\sigma_t}(x,\omega,t)\,\mathrm{d}t\,.$$

Using a change of variables, Lemma 6.3 and the mean value theorem for integration, we observe for both integrals

$$\int_{\tau_i-\Delta\tau_i}^{\tau_i} E_{\sigma_t}(x,\omega,t)\,\mathrm{d}t = \int_{-\Delta\tau_i}^{0} E_{\sigma_t}(x,\omega,\tau_i+t)\,\mathrm{d}t$$
$$= \int_{-\frac{h_\nu(p_i)}{\omega\cdot\nu(p_i)}}^{0} E_{\sigma_t}(x,\omega,\tau_i+t)\,\mathrm{d}t + o\big(\|h_\nu\|_{C^1}\big)$$
$$= E_{\sigma_t}(x,\omega,\tau_i+\widetilde{t}_i)\frac{h_\nu(p_i)}{\omega\cdot\nu(p_i)} + o\big(\|h_\nu\|_{C^1}\big)$$

---

[3]Recall $\frac{\mathrm{d}}{\mathrm{d}x}\int_0^{a(x)} f(t)\,\mathrm{d}t\Big|_{x=x_0} = f(a(x_0))a'(x_0)$.

for a $\tilde{t}_i \in \left]-\frac{h_\nu(p_i)}{\omega \cdot \nu(p_i)}, 0\right[$. Since $\psi(x, \omega) = 1$ and $x \notin \overline{\Gamma}$, the term $H(x, \omega)$ has the form

$$H(x, \omega) = -E_{\sigma_t}(x, \omega, \tau_1) \frac{h_\nu(p_1)}{\omega \cdot \nu(p_1)} + E_{\sigma_t}(x, \omega, \tau_2) \frac{h_\nu(p_2)}{\omega \cdot \nu(p_2)} .$$

It follows that

$$\frac{1}{\|h_\nu\|_{C^1}} \left| f_h(x, \omega) - f(x, \omega) - H(x, \omega) \right|$$

$$= \frac{1}{\|h_\nu\|_{C^1}} \left| \left(E_{\sigma_t}(x, \omega, \tau_1) - E_{\sigma_t}(x, \omega, \tau_1 + \tilde{t}_1) \right) \frac{h_\nu(p_1)}{\omega \cdot \nu(p_1)} \right.$$

$$\left. + \left(E_{\sigma_t}(x, \omega, \tau_2 + \tilde{t}_2) - E_{\sigma_t}(x, \omega, \tau_2) \right) \frac{h_\nu(p_2)}{\omega \cdot \nu(p_2)} \right| + o(1)$$

as $h \to 0$. In view of $\tilde{t}_i \in \left]-\frac{h_\nu(p_i)}{\omega \cdot \nu(p_i)}, 0\right[$ and of the continuity of $E_{\sigma_t}(x, \omega, \cdot)$, we obtain

$$\frac{1}{\|h_\nu\|_{C^1}} \left| f_h(x, \omega) - f(x, \omega) - H(x, \omega) \right| \to 0 \quad \text{as } h \to 0 .$$

Case $x \in \Gamma$:
We have for h sufficiently small that $\tau_2 - \Delta\tau_2 < 0$, i.e., $x \in \Gamma_h$. Thus, for h sufficiently small holds

$$f_h(x, \omega) - f(x, \omega) = \int_{\tau_1}^{\tau_1 - \Delta\tau_1} E_{\sigma_t}(x, \omega, t) \, dt$$

$$= -\int_{-\frac{h_\nu(p_1)}{\omega \cdot \nu(p_1)}}^{0} E_{\sigma_t}(x, \omega, \tau_1 + t) \, dt + o\big(\|h_\nu\|_{C^1}\big)$$

$$= -E_{\sigma_t}(x, \omega, \tau_1 + \tilde{t}) \frac{h_\nu(p_1)}{\omega \cdot \nu(p_1)} + o\big(\|h_\nu\|_{C^1}\big)$$

for a $\tilde{t} \in \left]-\frac{h_\nu(p_1)}{\omega \cdot \nu(p_1)}, 0\right[$. Since

$$H(x, \omega) = -E_{\sigma_t}(x, \omega, \tau_1) \frac{h_\nu(p_1)}{\omega \cdot \nu(p_1)}$$

for $x \in \Gamma$, we observe similar to the first case

$$\frac{1}{\|h_\nu\|_{C^1}} \left| f_h(x, \omega) - f(x, \omega) - H(x, \omega) \right| \to 0 \quad \text{as } h \to 0 .$$

Case $\psi(x, \omega) = 0$ and $x \notin \overline{\Gamma}$:
Then for h sufficiently small, $x \notin \Gamma_h$ and $\psi_h(x, \omega) = 0$. Hence, $f(x, \omega) = f_h(x, \omega) = 0 = H(x, \omega)$ when h is small.

Otherwise:
The other case, i.e., $x \in \partial\Gamma$, is irrelevant, as it only occurs for a subset of $X \times \Omega$ of measure zero.

We summarize that function H, defined in (6.17), is the pointwise domain derivative of the function f, that is, the asymptotic behavior

$$\frac{1}{\|h_\nu\|_{C^1}} |f_h(x,\omega) - f(x,\omega) - H(x,\omega)| \to 0 \quad \text{as } h \to 0$$

holds for almost all $(x,\omega) \in X \times \Omega$. $\qquad\square$

Remark 6.5. The function H can formally be seen as the 'solution' of the transmission boundary value problem

$$\omega \cdot \nabla H + \sigma_t H = h_\nu \delta|_{\partial\Gamma} \quad \text{in } X \times \Omega,$$
$$H = 0 \quad \text{on } \partial_-(X \times \Omega),$$

where $\delta|_{\partial\Gamma}$ is the delta distribution on $\partial\Gamma$. Actually, we have expected such an interpretation given the formal domain derivative in (6.4).

Let us verify this assertion: First, we observe that $h_\nu \delta|_{\partial\Gamma}$ coincides with

$$(y - t\omega, \omega) \mapsto \frac{h_\nu(y - t\omega)}{\omega \cdot \nu(y - t\omega)} \Big(\delta\big(t - \tau_2(y,\omega)\big) - \delta\big(t - \tau_1(y,\omega)\big) \Big)$$

as distribution on $X \times \Omega$, where for $\omega \in \Omega$ the elements of X are described by $y - t\omega$ with $y \in \partial X_{\omega,+}$ and $t \in]0, \tau_-(y,\omega)[$. This observation is due to a change of variable result akin to Lemma 2.1. From (2.24) we recall that $\mathcal{P}$ is the solution operator of the transport equation without scattering. Applying formally $\mathcal{P}$ to above distribution yields the statement.

6.2.3. Properties of the Function H. In this section we analyze the pointwise domain derivative H. We show that H lies in $L^1(X \times \Omega)$ and that its directional derivative $\omega \cdot \nabla H$ exists almost everywhere in $(X \setminus \overline{\Gamma}) \times \Omega$ and is even an element of $L^1((X \setminus \overline{\Gamma}) \times \Omega)$. Moreover, we specify Remark 6.5 and see that $\omega \cdot \nabla H = -\sigma_t H$ in $(X \setminus \overline{\Gamma}) \times \Omega$. This subsection will be completed by a trace theorem for a class of functions containing H. These results are used in the upcoming section to show that H is not only the pointwise but also the usual domain derivative of $\widetilde{F}$.

Theorem 6.6. *The function H defined in* (6.17) *is an element of* $L^1(X \times \Omega)$. *Moreover, there exists a constant $C > 0$ independent of h such that*

$$\|H\|_{L^1} \le C\|h_\nu\|_\infty.$$

PROOF. We only prove the theorem for $d = 3$ at this point, since it is the more relevant case in practice. The adaptions of the proof to the case $d = 2$ are presented in the Appendix C.0.1.

For $x \in X \setminus \partial\Gamma$ we define the absolute moment

$$\overline{H}(x) = \int_\Omega |H(x,\omega)| \, d\omega \, .$$

In the first step, we show that $\overline{H} \in L^1(\Gamma)$ and, in the second, that $\overline{H} \in L^1(X \setminus \overline{\Gamma})$. Then, the statement follows immediately.

Let $x \in \Gamma = B_R(0)$. In this case

$$H(x,\omega) = -E_{\sigma_t}\big(x,\omega,\tau_1(x,\omega)\big) \frac{h_\nu(p_1(x,\omega))}{\omega \cdot \nu(p_1(x,\omega))} \, .$$

Consequently,

$$\overline{H}(x) = \int_\Omega E_{\sigma_t}\big(x,\omega,\tau_1(x,\omega)\big) \frac{\big|h_\nu\big(p_1(x,\omega)\big)\big|}{\big|\omega \cdot \nu\big(p_1(x,\omega)\big)\big|} \, d\omega$$
$$\leq \|h_\nu\|_\infty \int_\Omega \frac{1}{\big|\omega \cdot \nu\big(p_1(x,\omega)\big)\big|} \, d\omega \, .$$

Before we calculate the latter integral, we simplify the expression in the denominator. As $\Gamma = B_R(0)$, the outer unit normal to Γ reads

$$\nu\big(p_1(x,\omega)\big) = \frac{1}{R} p_1(x,\omega) = \frac{1}{R}\big(x - \tau_1(x,\omega)\omega\big) \, .$$

Let $\omega_\perp \in \Omega$ be perpendicular to ω such that $x \cdot (\omega \times \omega_\perp) = 0$. Multiplying the normal by ω and inserting the representation (6.11) of τ_1, we get

$$\omega \cdot \nu\big(p_1(x,\omega)\big) = \frac{1}{R}\big(x - \tau_1(x,\omega)\omega\big) \cdot \omega$$
$$= \frac{1}{R}\big(-\sqrt{R^2 - (x^T\omega_\perp)^2}\,\omega + x^T\omega_\perp\,\omega_\perp\big) \cdot \omega$$
$$= -\frac{1}{R}\sqrt{R^2 - (x^T\omega_\perp)^2} \, .$$

For $x \neq 0$ the integral can be calculated as follows

$$
\begin{aligned}
\int_{\Omega} \frac{1}{\left|\omega \cdot \nu\big(p_1(x,\omega)\big)\right|}\, \mathrm{d}\omega &= R \int_{\Omega} \frac{1}{\sqrt{R^2 - (x^T \omega_\perp)^2}}\, \mathrm{d}\omega \\
&= \frac{R}{|x|} \int_{\Omega} \left(\frac{R^2}{|x|^2} - \left(\left(\frac{x}{|x|} \right)^T \omega_\perp \right)^2 \right)^{-\frac{1}{2}} \mathrm{d}\omega_\perp \\
&= 2\pi \frac{R}{|x|} \int_{-1}^{1} \left(\frac{R^2}{|x|^2} - s^2 \right)^{-\frac{1}{2}} \mathrm{d}s \qquad\qquad (6.18) \\
&= 2\pi \frac{R}{|x|} \arcsin\!\left(\frac{s|x|}{R} \right) \Bigg|_{-1}^{1} \\
&= 4\pi \frac{R}{|x|} \arcsin\!\left(\frac{|x|}{R} \right),
\end{aligned}
$$

where we use in the third equation the change of variable $s = x^T \omega_\perp / |x|$, see Section VII.2 in [**Nat01b**] for more details. For $x = 0$ holds

$$
\int_{\Omega} \frac{1}{\left|\omega \cdot \nu\big(p_1(0,\omega)\big)\right|}\, \mathrm{d}\omega = \int_{\Omega} 1\, \mathrm{d}\omega = 4\pi\,.
$$

The right-hand side of the last equation coincides with the limit of $4\pi \arcsin(s)/s$ as $s \to 0+$. This function is monotone increasing on $[0,1]$ and the upper bound is $4\pi \arcsin 1 = 2\pi^2$. Thus,

$$
\overline{H}|_{\Gamma} \in L^{\infty}(\Gamma) \subset L^1(\Gamma) \quad \text{with} \quad \|\overline{H}|_{\Gamma}\|_{\infty} \le 2\pi^2 \|h_\nu\|_{\infty}
$$

and

$$
H|_{\Gamma \times \Omega} \in L^1(\Gamma \times \Omega)\,.
$$

Let now $x \in X \setminus \overline{\Gamma}$. Then, $x \in X$ with $|x| > R$. We consider again $\overline{H}$ and observe that directions with $\psi(x,\omega) = 0$ have no influence on the value of $\overline{H}(x)$, where ψ is the visibility function defined in (6.8). We recall the equivalence (6.9) for $x \notin \overline{\Gamma}$:

$$
\psi(x,\omega) = 1 \iff x^T \omega > 0 \text{ and } x^T \omega_\perp \in \,]{-R},R[\,.
$$

Using the visibility function, we rewrite

$$
\begin{aligned}
\overline{H}(x) = \int_{\Omega} \psi(x,\omega) \Bigg| & E_{\sigma_t}\big(x,\omega,\tau_2(x,\omega)\big) \frac{h_\nu(p_2(x,\omega))}{\omega \cdot \nu(p_2(x,\omega))} \\
& - E_{\sigma_t}\big(x,\omega,\tau_1(x,\omega)\big) \frac{h_\nu(p_1(x,\omega))}{\omega \cdot \nu(p_1(x,\omega))} \Bigg|\, \mathrm{d}\omega
\end{aligned}
$$

and immediately obtain the estimate

$$\overline{H}(x) \leq \|h_\nu\|_\infty \int_\Omega \psi(x,\omega) \left(\frac{1}{|\omega \cdot \nu(p_2(x,\omega))|} + \frac{1}{|\omega \cdot \nu(p_1(x,\omega))|} \right) d\omega \,.$$

Only the ω with $\psi(x,\omega) = 1$ have an impact on the integral on the right-hand side. Given such an ω, we have the representation

$$p_i(x,\omega) = x^T \omega_\perp \, \omega_\perp + (-1)^i \sqrt{R^2 - (x^T \omega_\perp)^2} \, \omega$$

for $i = 1, 2$, recalling (6.10). Multiplying this identity with ω and using the form of the normal vector, yields

$$\omega \cdot \nu(p_i(x,\omega)) = \frac{1}{R} p_i(x,\omega) \cdot \omega = (-1)^i \frac{1}{R} \sqrt{R^2 - (x^T \omega_\perp)^2} \,.$$

Thus, the two integrals in the estimate of $\overline{H}$ can be rewritten as

$$\int_\Omega \frac{\psi(x,\omega)}{|\omega \cdot \nu(p_i(x,\omega))|} \, d\omega = R \int_{x^T \omega_\perp \in]-R,R[} \frac{1}{\sqrt{R^2 - (x^T \omega_\perp)^2}} \, d\omega_\perp \,.$$

Using a parameterization $\omega_\perp(\phi, \vartheta)$ of the sphere Ω such that $x^T \omega_\perp = |x| \cos \vartheta$, i.e., the 'usual' parameterization with $x/|x|$ as north pole, we obtain by two changes of variables

$$R \int_{x^T \omega_\perp \in]-R,R[} \frac{1}{\sqrt{R^2 - (x^T \omega_\perp)^2}} \, d\omega_\perp$$

$$= R \int_{\arccos(\frac{R}{|x|})}^{\arccos(-\frac{R}{|x|})} \int_0^{2\pi} \frac{1}{\sqrt{R^2 - (|x| \cos \vartheta)^2}} \sin \vartheta \, d\phi \, d\vartheta$$

$$= 2\pi R \int_{-\frac{R}{|x|}}^{\frac{R}{|x|}} \frac{1}{\sqrt{R^2 - |x|^2 s^2}} \, ds \qquad (6.19)$$

$$= 2\pi \frac{R}{|x|} \arcsin\left(\frac{s|x|}{R}\right) \Bigg|_{-\frac{R}{|x|}}^{\frac{R}{|x|}}$$

$$= 2\pi^2 \frac{R}{|x|} \,.$$

This term is obviously bounded by $2\pi^2$ on $X \setminus \overline{\Gamma} = X \setminus \overline{B_R(0)}$. Thus,

$$\overline{H} \in L^\infty(X \setminus \overline{\Gamma}) \subset L^1(X \setminus \overline{\Gamma}) \,.$$

This implies

$$H|_{(X \setminus \overline{\Gamma}) \times \Omega} \in L^1\big((X \setminus \overline{\Gamma}) \times \Omega\big) \,.$$

Combining the two developed estimates

$$\|\overline{H}|_\Gamma\|_\infty \le 2\pi^2\|h_\nu\|_\infty \quad \text{and} \quad \|\overline{H}|_{X\setminus\overline{\Gamma}}\|_\infty \le 4\pi^2\|h_\nu\|_\infty\,,$$

we finally observe

$$H \in L^1(X \times \Omega) \quad \text{with} \quad \|H\|_{L^1} \le 4\pi^2\mathrm{Vol}(X)\|h_\nu\|_\infty\,.$$

$\square$

Remark 6.7. The result of Theorem 6.6 cannot be generalized to L^p spaces with $p \ge 2$. Proceeding as in the previous proof, we would have to integrate $1-s^2$ instead of $\sqrt{1-s^2}$. But the former function, its primitive is Artanh, is not integrable over the interval $[-1,1]$. We obtain for constant h_ν a lower bound of $\overline{H}(x)$ that is unbounded for all $x \in X \setminus \overline{\Gamma}$.

The function H is not only in $L^1(X \times \Omega)$, but also its directional derivative $\omega \cdot \nabla H$ exists in $L^1\big((X \setminus \overline{\Gamma}) \times \Omega\big)$.

Lemma 6.8. *The directional derivative $\omega \cdot \nabla H$ of the function H, defined in (6.17), exists almost everywhere in $(X\setminus\overline{\Gamma})\times\Omega$ and lies in $L^1\big((X\setminus\overline{\Gamma})\times\Omega\big)$. Moreover, the identity*

$$\omega \cdot \nabla H(x,\omega) = -\sigma_{\mathrm{t}}(x)H(x,\omega)$$

holds for almost all $(x,\omega) \in (X \setminus \overline{\Gamma}) \times \Omega$.

PROOF. For $x \in X \setminus \overline{\Gamma}$ and $\omega \in \Omega$ the function H admits the form

$$H(x,\omega) = \psi(x,\omega) \sum_{i=1}^{2} (-1)^i E_{\sigma_{\mathrm{t}}}\big(x,\omega,\tau_i(x,\omega)\big)\frac{h_\nu(p_i(x,\omega))}{\omega \cdot \nu(p_i(x,\omega))}\,.$$

Moreover, we have for $(x,\omega) \in (X \setminus \overline{\Gamma}) \times \Omega$ and t sufficiently small:

$$\psi(x + t\omega,\omega) = \psi(x,\omega)\,,$$

$$\tau_i(x + t\omega,\omega) = (x + t\omega)^T\omega - (-1)^i\sqrt{R^2 - \big((x + t\omega)^T\omega_\perp\big)^2} = t + \tau_i(x,\omega)\,,$$

$$p_i(x + t\omega,\omega) = x + t\omega - \tau_i(x + t\omega,\omega)\omega = x - \tau_i(x,\omega)\omega = p_i(x,\omega)\,.$$

In other words, the intersection points of $l_{x,\omega}$ and Γ do not change under variations in direction ω (unless $x + t\omega \in \Gamma$); only the travel time to the intersection point changes in an identical way.

Thus, the function $E_{\sigma_{\mathrm{t}}}$ is the sole term in H effected by a variation of x in direction ω. It suffices to calculate the directional derivative of $E_{\sigma_{\mathrm{t}}}$.

By the chain rule we obtain

$$
\frac{\partial}{\partial t} E_{\sigma_t}\big(x + t\omega, \omega, \tau_i(x + t\omega, \omega)\big)\Big|_{t=0} = \frac{\partial}{\partial t} \exp\left(-\int_{-t}^{\tau_i(x,\omega)} \sigma_t(x - s\omega)\,ds\right)\Big|_{t=0}
$$

$$
= -\sigma_t(x) E_{\sigma_t}\big(x, \omega, \tau_i(x, \omega)\big)
$$

for almost all $(x, \omega) \in (X \setminus \overline{\Gamma}) \times \Omega$.

Using the relation (2.19) for the directional derivative and combining the identities developed above, we conclude

$$
\omega \cdot \nabla H(x, \omega) = \frac{\partial}{\partial t} H(x + t\omega, \omega)\Big|_{t=0}
$$

$$
= \psi(x, \omega) \sum_{i=1}^{2} (-1)^{i+1} \sigma_t(x) E_{\sigma_t}\big(x, \omega, \tau_i(x, \omega)\big) \frac{h_\nu(p_i(x, \omega))}{\omega \cdot \nu(p_i(x, \omega))}
$$

$$
= -\sigma_t(x) H(x, \omega)
$$

for almost all $(x, \omega) \in (X \setminus \overline{\Gamma}) \times \Omega$. Since $H \in L^1(X \times \Omega)$ and $\sigma_t \in L^\infty(X)$, the directional derivative $\omega \cdot \nabla H$ particularly lies in $L^1\big((X \setminus \overline{\Gamma}) \times \Omega\big)$. $\square$

Later we also need a result on the trace of H. Since the trace theorems stated in Section 2.2.1 and other trace theorems from the literature[4] are not directly applicable, we develop the following result for a class of functions containing H. The argument is similar to the proof of the trace theorem stated in [**CS99**, Theorem 2.1], which coincides with Lemma 2.3 above. For the sake of convenience, we recall the definition of the space $\mathcal{Y}$, which contains the trace of H:

$$
\mathcal{Y} = L^1\big(\partial_+(X \times \Omega), |\omega \cdot \nu|\, d\mu\, d\omega\big),
$$

compare (6.1).

Lemma 6.9. *Let $M > 0$ such that $\overline{B_M(0)} \subset X$. Set $a_X = \mathrm{dist}(B_M(0), \partial X)$. Moreover, let $v \in L^1(X \times \Omega)$ with $\omega \cdot \nabla v \in L^1\big((X \setminus B_M(0)) \times \Omega\big)$ and $v(x, \omega) = 0$ if $l_{x,\omega} \cap B_M(0) = \emptyset$. Then,*

$$
\|\gamma_+ v\|_{\mathcal{Y}} \le \|\omega \cdot \nabla v\|_{L^1\big((X \setminus B_M(0)) \times \Omega\big)} + \frac{1}{a_X} \|v\|_{L^1\big((X \setminus B_M(0)) \times \Omega\big)},
$$

where $\gamma_+ v = v|_{\partial_+(X \times \Omega)}$.

PROOF. We set

$$
\varphi(t) = v(y - t\omega, \omega)
$$

for $(y, \omega) \in \partial_+(X \times \Omega)$ and $t \in \big[0, \min\{a_X, \tau_-(y, \omega)\}\big]$.

---

[4]At least those results we known.

If $\tau_-(y,\omega) \leq a_X$, then $\varphi(t) \equiv 0$ as $l_{x,\omega} \cap B_M(0) = \emptyset$. Thus, the estimate

$$|v(y,\omega)| \leq \int_0^{\tau_-(y,\omega)} |\omega \cdot \nabla v(y - s\omega, \omega)| \, ds + \frac{1}{a_X} \int_0^{\tau_-(y,\omega)} |v(y - s\omega, \omega)| \, ds$$

is trivial in this case.

Otherwise, we have by the mean value theorem

$$|\varphi(0)| \leq |\varphi(t)| + \int_0^t |\varphi'(s)| \, ds \leq |\varphi(t)| + \|\varphi'\|_{L^1(0,a_x)}$$

for all $t \in [0, a_X]$. By Integration of this estimate over the interval $[0, a_X]$ it follows that

$$|\varphi(0)| \leq \|\varphi'\|_{L^1(0,a_x)} + \frac{1}{a_X} \|\varphi\|_{L^1(0,a_x)} \, .$$

In terms of v the preceding formula becomes

$$|v(y,\omega)| \leq \int_0^{a_X} |\omega \cdot \nabla v(y - s\omega, \omega)| \, ds + \frac{1}{a_X} \int_0^{a_X} |v(y - s\omega, \omega)| \, ds$$

$$\leq \int_0^{|y|-M} |\omega \cdot \nabla v(y - s\omega, \omega)| \, ds + \frac{1}{a_X} \int_0^{|y|-M} |v(y - s\omega, \omega)| \, ds \, .$$

Integrating this estimate over $\partial_+(X \times \Omega)$ with respect to the measure $|\omega \cdot \nu| \, d\omega \, d\mu$ and using the change of variable rule from Lemma 2.1 adapted to $(X \setminus B_M(0)) \times \Omega$, we finally obtain

$$\|\gamma_+ v\|_{\mathcal{Y}} = \int_\Omega \int_{\partial X_{\omega,+}} |v(y,\omega)| |\omega \cdot \nu(y)| \, d\mu(y) \, d\omega$$

$$\leq \int_\Omega \int_{\partial X_{\omega,+}} \int_0^{\min\{\tau_-(y,\omega),|y|-M\}} |\omega \cdot \nabla v(y - t\omega, \omega)| |\omega \cdot \nu(y)| \, dt \, d\mu(y) \, d\omega$$

$$+ \int_\Omega \int_{\partial X_{\omega,+}} \int_0^{\min\{\tau_-(y,\omega),|y|-M\}} \frac{1}{a_X} |v(y - t\omega, \omega)| |\omega \cdot \nu(y)| \, dt \, d\mu(y) \, d\omega$$

$$\leq \int_{X \setminus B_M(0)} \int_\Omega |\omega \cdot \nabla v(x,\omega)| + \frac{1}{a_X} |v(x,\omega)| \, d\omega \, dx$$

$$= \|\omega \cdot \nabla v\|_{L^1\left((X \setminus B_M(0)) \times \Omega\right)} + \frac{1}{a_X} \|v\|_{L^1\left((X \setminus B_M(0)) \times \Omega\right)} \, .$$

$$\square$$

6.2.4. Domain Derivative of $\widetilde{F}$. Having the analysis of H finished, we now address the question of domain differentiability of $\widetilde{F}$. We see in the upcoming theorem that the function H is not only the pointwise domain derivative, but also the usual domain derivative.

Theorem 6.10. *It holds*

$$\lim_{h\to 0} \frac{1}{\|h_\nu\|_{C^1}} \|f_h - f - H\|_{L^1} = 0.$$

To prove this theorem, we use the dominated convergence theorem, see e.g. [**Lan93**]. The pointwise convergence of $|f_h - f - H|/\|h_\nu\|$ is developed in Theorem 6.4. The existence of an uniform, thus integrable, upper bound is a consequence of the following lemma together with Theorem 6.6.

Lemma 6.11. *The term*

$$\frac{1}{\|h_\nu\|_\infty} \|f_h - f\|_{L^1}$$

is uniformly bounded for all h with $\|h_\nu\|_\infty$ sufficiently small.

PROOF. We only prove the lemma for $d = 3$ here. The necessary adaptions to the case $d = 2$ are found in the Appendix C.0.2.

To show the statement, we split the L^1 norm into 3 parts, namely

$$\|f_h - f\|_{L^1}$$
$$\leq \|(f_h - f)\chi_{\Gamma \cap \Gamma_h}\|_{L^1} + \|(f_h - f)\chi_{X \setminus (\Gamma \cup \Gamma_h)}\|_{L^1} + \|(f_h - f)\chi_{\Gamma \Delta \Gamma_h}\|_{L^1}.$$

Herein, $\Gamma \Delta \Gamma_h$ denotes the symmetric difference of Γ and Γ_h, i.e., $\Gamma \Delta \Gamma_h = (\Gamma \setminus \Gamma_h) \cup (\Gamma_h \setminus \Gamma)$. The next and crucial part is to estimate each summand of the decomposition.

Before we start, let us recall a few results from above. The functions f and f_h admit the representations

$$f(x,\omega) = \psi(x,\omega) \int_{\max\{0,\tau_2(x,\omega)\}}^{\tau_1(x,\omega)} E_{\sigma_t}(x,\omega,t)\,\mathrm{d}t,$$

$$f_h(x,\omega) = \psi_h(x,\omega) \int_{\max\{0,\tau_2^h(x,\omega)\}}^{\tau_1^h(x,\omega)} E_{\sigma_t}(x,\omega,t)\,\mathrm{d}t,$$

compare (6.15) and (6.16). From Lemma 6.2 we know that

$$|\Delta\tau_i| = |\tau_i^h(x,\omega) - \tau_i(x,\omega)| \leq \frac{3\|h_\nu\|_\infty}{|\omega \cdot \nu(p_i(x,\omega))|}$$

for $i = 1, 2$ if $\psi(x,\omega) = \psi_h(x,\omega) = 1$. In addition, it is shown in the proof of Theorem 6.6 that the product of $\psi(x,\omega)$ and the right-hand side of the last estimate is integrable over Ω with

$$3\|h_\nu\|_\infty \int_\Omega \psi(x,\omega) \frac{1}{|\omega \cdot \nu(p_i(x,\omega))|}\, d\omega \leq 6\pi^2 \|h_\nu\|_\infty \qquad (6.20)$$

for $x \in X \setminus \partial\Gamma$.

Now we estimate each of the three summands:

$\|(f_h - f)\chi_{\Gamma \cap \Gamma_h}\|_{L^1}$:

For all $x \in \Gamma \cap \Gamma_h$ holds $\psi(x,\cdot) = \psi_h(x,\cdot) = 1$. Hence,

$$\begin{aligned}
\|(f_h - f)\chi_{\Gamma \cap \Gamma_h}\|_{L^1} &= \int_{\Gamma \cap \Gamma_h} \int_\Omega \left| \int_{\tau_1(x,\omega)}^{\tau_1^h(x,\omega)} E_{\sigma_t}(x,\omega,t)\, dt \right| d\omega\, dx \\
&\leq \int_{\Gamma \cap \Gamma_h} \int_\Omega |\Delta\tau_1(x,\omega)|\, d\omega\, dx \\
&\leq 3\|h_\nu\|_\infty \int_\Gamma \int_\Omega \frac{1}{|\omega \cdot \nu(p_1(x,\omega))|}\, d\omega\, dx
\end{aligned}$$

Using (6.20) and $\mathrm{Vol}(\Gamma) = 4\pi R^3/3$, we obtain

$$\|(f_h - f)\chi_{\Gamma \cap \Gamma_h}\|_{L^1} \leq 8\pi^3 R^3 \|h_\nu\|_\infty = C_1 \|h_\nu\|_\infty . \qquad (6.21)$$

$\|(f_h - f)\chi_{\Gamma \Delta \Gamma_h}\|_{L^1}$:

Obviously, $\Gamma \Delta \Gamma_h \subset B_{R+\|h_\nu\|_\infty}(0) \setminus B_{R-\|h_\nu\|_\infty}(0)$ holds. Thus,

$$\|\chi_{\Gamma \Delta \Gamma_h}\|_{L^1} = \mathrm{Vol}(\Gamma \Delta \Gamma_h) \leq \frac{8}{3}\pi\big(3R^2 + \|h_\nu\|_\infty^2\big)\|h_\nu\|_\infty .$$

Moreover, the functions f and f_h are bounded with

$$\|f\|_\infty \leq 2R \quad \text{and} \quad \|f_h\|_\infty \leq 2\big(R + \|h_\nu\|_\infty\big),$$

since the length of the intersection $l_{x,\omega} \cap \Gamma$ and $l_{x,\omega} \cap \Gamma_h$ is maximal the diameter of Γ and Γ_h, respectively. It follows that

$$\begin{aligned}
\|(f_h - f)\chi_{\Gamma \Delta \Gamma_h}\|_{L^1} &\leq \|f_h \chi_{\Gamma \Delta \Gamma_h}\|_{L^1} + \|f \chi_{\Gamma \Delta \Gamma_h}\|_{L^1} \\
&\leq \frac{16}{3}\pi\big(3R^2 + \|h_\nu\|_\infty^2\big)\big(2R + \|h_\nu\|_\infty\big)\|h_\nu\|_\infty .
\end{aligned}$$

So we can find a constant $C_2 > 0$ such that

$$\|(f_h - f)\chi_{\Gamma \Delta \Gamma_h}\|_{L^1} \leq C_2 \|h_\nu\|_\infty$$

for all h sufficiently small.

$\|(f_h - f)\chi_{X \setminus (\Gamma \cup \Gamma_h)}\|_{L^1}$:

Let $x \in X \setminus (\overline{\Gamma \cup \Gamma_h})$. We define $\overline{\Delta f}(x)$ as the absolute moment of $f_h(x,\cdot) - f(x,\cdot)$, that is,

$$\overline{\Delta f}(x) = \int_\Omega |f_h(x,\omega) - f(x,\omega)|\, d\omega .$$

Since $f_h(x, \cdot) - f(x, \cdot) = 0$ if $\big(1 - \psi_h(x, \cdot)\big)\big(1 - \psi(x, \cdot)\big) \neq 0$, the moment $\overline{\Delta f}(x)$ can be written as

$$
\begin{aligned}
\overline{\Delta f}(x) = &\int_{\Omega} \psi(x, \omega)\psi_h(x, \omega)\big|f_h(x, \omega) - f(x, \omega)\big|\, d\omega \\
&+ \int_{\Omega} \psi(x, \omega)\big(1 - \psi_h(x, \omega)\big)\big|f_h(x, \omega) - f(x, \omega)\big|\, d\omega \qquad (6.22) \\
&+ \int_{\Omega} \big(1 - \psi(x, \omega)\big)\psi_h(x, \omega)\big|f_h(x, \omega) - f(x, \omega)\big|\, d\omega\,.
\end{aligned}
$$

We consider each of the integrals in (6.22) separately, in order to show the uniform boundedness of $\|(f_h - f)\chi_{X\setminus(\Gamma\cup\Gamma_h)}\|_{L^1}$.

The first integral in (6.22) can be estimated as follows:

$$
\begin{aligned}
&\int_{\Omega} \psi(x, \omega)\psi_h(x, \omega)\big|f_h(x, \omega) - f(x, \omega)\big|\, d\omega \\
&= \int_{\Omega} \psi(x, \omega)\psi_h(x, \omega)\bigg|\sum_{i=1}^{2}(-1)^i \int_{\tau_i^h(x,\omega)}^{\tau_i(x,\omega)} E_{\sigma_t}(x, \omega, t)\, dt\bigg|\, d\omega \\
&\leq 3\|h_\nu\|_\infty \int_{\Omega} \psi(x, \omega)\psi_h(x, \omega)\bigg(\frac{1}{|\omega \cdot \nu\big(p_1(x,\omega)\big)|} + \frac{1}{|\omega \cdot \nu\big(p_2(x,\omega)\big)|}\bigg)\, d\omega \\
&\leq 12\pi^2\|h_\nu\|_\infty\,, \qquad\qquad\qquad\qquad\qquad\qquad\qquad\qquad\qquad\qquad (6.23)
\end{aligned}
$$

where we again use (6.20) in the last step.

Before estimating the second integral in (6.22), we observe that, according to (6.9) and its perturbed variant, $\psi(x, \omega) = 1$ and $\psi_h(x, \omega) = 0$ imply

$$
R - \|h_\nu\|_\infty \leq |x^T\omega_\perp| < R\,.
$$

It follows that

$$
\begin{aligned}
|\tau_2(x, \omega) - \tau_1(x, \omega)| &= 2\sqrt{R^2 - (x^T\omega_\perp)^2} \\
&\leq 2\sqrt{R^2 - \big(R - \|h_\nu\|_\infty\big)^2} = 2\sqrt{2\|h_\nu\|_\infty R - \|h_\nu\|_\infty^2}
\end{aligned}
$$

if $\psi(x, \omega) = 1$ and $\psi_h(x, \omega) = 0$. Moreover, we know from (6.16) that $f_h(x, \omega)$ vanishes if $\psi_h(x, \omega)$ does. Taking these observations into account, we obtain

$$
\int_\Omega \psi(x,\omega)\big(1 - \psi_h(x,\omega)\big)\big|f_h(x,\omega) - f(x,\omega)\big|\,\mathrm{d}\omega
$$

$$
= \int_\Omega \psi(x,\omega)\big(1 - \psi_h(x,\omega)\big)\big|f(x,\omega)\big|\,\mathrm{d}\omega
$$

$$
= \int_\Omega \psi(x,\omega)\big(1 - \psi_h(x,\omega)\big)\left|\int_{\tau_2(x,\omega)}^{\tau_1(x,\omega)} E_{\sigma_t}(x,\omega,t)\right|\,\mathrm{d}\omega
$$

$$
\leq \int_\Omega \psi(x,\omega)\big(1 - \psi_h(x,\omega)\big)\big|\tau_1(x,\omega) - \tau_2(x,\omega)\big|\,\mathrm{d}\omega
$$

$$
\leq \int_{|x^T\omega_\perp|\in[R-\|h_\nu\|_\infty,R[} 2\sqrt{2\|h_\nu\|_\infty R - \|h_\nu\|_\infty^2}\,\mathrm{d}\omega \tag{6.24}
$$

$$
= 4\sqrt{2\|h_\nu\|_\infty R - \|h_\nu\|_\infty^2}\int_{x^T\omega_\perp\in[R-\|h_\nu\|_\infty,R[} 1\,\mathrm{d}\omega_\perp
$$

$$
= 4\sqrt{2\|h_\nu\|_\infty R - \|h_\nu\|_\infty^2}\int_0^{2\pi}\int_{\arccos(\frac{R}{|x|})}^{\arccos(\frac{R-\|h_\nu\|_\infty}{|x|})} \sin\vartheta\,\mathrm{d}\vartheta\,\mathrm{d}\phi
$$

$$
= 8\pi\sqrt{2\|h_\nu\|_\infty R - \|h_\nu\|_\infty^2}\int_{\frac{R-\|h_\nu\|_\infty}{|x|}}^{\frac{R}{|x|}} 1\,\mathrm{d}s
$$

$$
\leq \frac{8\pi}{R}\|h_\nu\|_\infty^{\frac{3}{2}}\sqrt{2R - \|h_\nu\|_\infty}\,.
$$

In order to estimate the third integral in (6.22), we make similar observations: If $\psi(x,\omega) = 0$ and $\psi_h(x,\omega) = 1$ holds, then

$$
R \leq |x^T\omega_\perp| < R + \|h_\nu\|_\infty\,.
$$

For such ω we have, moreover, that

$$
|\tau_2^h(x,\omega) - \tau_1^h(x,\omega)| \leq 2\sqrt{(R + \|h_\nu\|_\infty)^2 - (x^T\omega_\perp)^2}
$$

$$
\leq 2\sqrt{2R\|h_\nu\|_\infty + \|h_\nu\|_\infty^2}
$$

and $f(x,\omega) = 0$. By similar arguments as above, it follows that

$$\int_\Omega \big(1 - \psi(x,\omega)\big)\psi_h(x,\omega)\big|f_h(x,\omega) - f(x,\omega)\big|\,\mathrm{d}\omega$$

$$\leq \int_\Omega \big(1 - \psi(x,\omega)\big)\psi_h(x,\omega)\big|\tau_1^h(x,\omega) - \tau_2^h(x,\omega)\big|\,\mathrm{d}\omega$$

$$\leq 4\sqrt{2R\|h_\nu\|_\infty + \|h_\nu\|_\infty^2}\int_{x^T\omega_\perp \in [R,R+\|h_\nu\|_\infty[} 1\,\mathrm{d}\omega_\perp$$

$$= 8\pi\sqrt{2R\|h_\nu\|_\infty + \|h_\nu\|_\infty^2}\int_{\frac{R}{|x|}}^{\frac{R+\|h_\nu\|_\infty}{|x|}} 1\,\mathrm{d}s$$

$$= \frac{8\pi}{R}\|h_\nu\|_\infty^{\frac{3}{2}}\sqrt{2R + \|h_\nu\|_\infty}\,. \tag{6.25}$$

We merge the estimates of the three summands in (6.22) and conclude that there is a constant $C_3 > 0$ such that

$$\|(f_h - f)\chi_{X\setminus(\Gamma\cup\Gamma_h)}\|_{L^1} \leq \|\overline{\Delta f}\|_\infty \mathrm{Vol}(\Gamma) \leq C_3\|h_\nu\|_\infty$$

for all h sufficiently small.

Finally, we add up all spatial parts of the L^1 norm of $f_h - f$ to obtain

$$\|f_h - f\|_{L^1} \leq (C_1 + C_2 + C_3)\|h_\nu\|_\infty$$

for all h sufficiently small. $\qquad\square$

Corollary 6.12. *There exists an $M > 0$ such that*

$$\frac{1}{\|h_\nu\|_\infty}\|f_h - f - H\|_{L^1} \leq M$$

for all h sufficiently small.

PROOF. From Theorem 6.6 we know that there is a constant $C > 0$ with

$$\|H\|_{L^1} \leq C\|h_\nu\|_\infty\,.$$

By the triangle equality and Lemma 6.11 the statements follows. $\qquad\square$

PROOF OF THEOREM 6.10. In Theorem 6.4 the pointwise convergence, $\frac{1}{\|h_\nu\|_{C^1}}|f_h - f - H| \to 0$ almost everywhere in $X \times \Omega$ as $h \to 0$, is established. In Corollary 6.12 it is shown that the L^1 norm of these functions are uniformly bounded for h sufficiently small. As $X \times \Omega$ is bounded, the statement is an immediate consequence of the dominated convergence theorem. $\qquad\square$

6.2.5. Domain Derivative of $\gamma_+\widetilde{F}$. Although we have now all ingredients at hand to calculate the domain derivative of F directly, we do an intermediate step here. We consider the special case of purely absorbing media, i.e., $\sigma_s = 0$ and $\mathcal{K} = 0$. Since it is the framework of SPECT, it is of special interest.[5]

Theorem 6.13. *The domain derivative of $\gamma_+\widetilde{F}(\Gamma)$ is the trace $\gamma_+ H$ of the function H defined in (6.17), that is,*

$$\frac{1}{\|h_\nu\|_{C^1}}\|\gamma_+(f_h - f - H)\|_{\mathcal{Y}} \to 0 \quad as \ h \to 0.$$

PROOF. Let $M > 0$ be such that $\overline{\Gamma \cup \Gamma_h} \subset \overline{B_M(0)} \subset X$. We recall that f and f_h are the solutions of $(\omega \cdot \nabla + \sigma_t I)f = \chi_\Gamma$ and $(\omega \cdot \nabla + \sigma_t I)f_h = \chi_{\Gamma_h}$, respectively. From Lemma 6.8 we know that $(\omega \cdot \nabla + \sigma_t)H = 0$ on $X \setminus \overline{\Gamma}$. Consequently,

$$\omega \cdot \nabla(f_h - f - H) = \sigma_t(H + f - f_h) \quad \text{in } (X \setminus \overline{B_M(0)}) \times \Omega$$

and

$$\|\omega \cdot \nabla(f_h - f - H)\|_{L^1\left((X\setminus\overline{B_M(0)})\times\Omega\right)} \le \|\sigma_t\|_\infty\|f_h - f - H\|_{L^1}.$$

So, the function $f_h - f - H$ fulfills the conditions of Lemma 6.9, which states that trace of $f_h - f - H$ satisfies

$$\|\gamma_+(f_h - f - H)\|_{\mathcal{Y}} \le \left(\|\sigma_t\|_\infty + \frac{1}{a_X}\right)\|f_h - f - H\|_{L^1}$$

with $a_X = \text{dist}(B_M(0), X)$. In view of Theorem 6.10, the statement follows immediately. $\qquad\square$

Remark 6.14. Since the integral operator $\mathcal{P}$, defined in (2.23), and the attenuated ray transform P_{σ_t} coincide up to notation and since the norm identity (2.26) holds, we directly obtain the domain derivative of the operator

$$P_{\sigma_t} \circ Q \colon \mathcal{S} \to L^1(T), \quad P_{\sigma_t} \circ Q(G) = \lambda P_{\sigma_t}\chi_G$$

about a ball Γ:

$$\left((P_{\sigma_t} \circ Q)'(\Gamma)h\right)(y,\omega) = \lambda \int_{\mathbb{R}} \exp\left(-\int_t^\infty \sigma_t(y + s\omega)\,\mathrm{d}s\right) \frac{h_\nu(y + t\omega)}{\omega \cdot \nu(y + t\omega)}$$
$$\left(\delta\big(t + \tau_2(y,\omega)\big) - \delta\big(t + \tau_1(y,\omega)\big)\right)\mathrm{d}t$$

---

[5]We are not aware of a result concerning the domain derivative of the SPECT forward operator.

for $(y, \omega) \in T$. Herein, $\mathcal{S}$ is the set of smooth domains and T the tangent bundle of Ω, i.e., $T = \{(x, \theta) \in \mathbb{R}^d \times \Omega \colon x \in \theta^\perp\}$.

We note that a similar result is developed in Appendix E for general convex domains, but only in case $d = 2$ and in a negative order Sobolev space.

6.2.6. Domain Derivative of F. Finally, we state the main result of this section, namely a theorem characterizing the domain derivative of F about a ball.

Theorem 6.15. *The domain derivative of F about the ball $\Gamma = B_R(0)$ in direction $h \in C_0^1(X, \mathbb{R}^d)$ is given by*

$$F'(\lambda, \Gamma)h = \lambda \gamma_+ (I + L^{-1}S)H,$$

where γ_+ is the trace operator, L the transport operator given in (2.21), S the scattering operator introduced in (2.4) and H the function defined in (6.17).

PROOF. The forward operator F can be decomposed as

$$F(\lambda, \cdot) = \lambda \gamma_+ (I - \mathcal{K})^{-1}\widetilde{F} = \lambda \gamma_+ (I + L^{-1}S)\widetilde{F},$$

as seen in (6.5) and Lemma 6.1. In Theorem 6.10 and 6.13 we have seen that H and $\gamma_+ H$ are the domain derivatives of $\widetilde{F}$ and of $\gamma_+ \widetilde{F}$, respectively. Hence,

$$\frac{1}{\|h_\nu\|_{C^1}}\|(f_h - f - H)\|_{L^1} \to 0 \quad \text{and} \quad \frac{1}{\|h_\nu\|_{C^1}}\|\gamma_+(f_h - f - H)\|_{\mathcal{Y}} \to 0$$

hold as $h \to 0$.

Moreover, the operator $\gamma_+ L^{-1}S$ is a bounded linear operator from $L^1(X \times \Omega)$ to $\mathcal{Y}$. This is the case, as it is the composition of the bounded linear operators $S \colon L^1(X \times \Omega) \to L^1(X \times \Omega)$, $L^{-1} \colon L^1(X \times \Omega) \to W_-^1(X \times \Omega)$ and $\gamma_+ \colon W_-^1(X \times \Omega) \to \mathcal{Y}$. The continuity of the latter two operators is addressed in Corollary 2.5 and Lemma 2.3.

Consequently,

$$\frac{1}{\|h_\nu\|_{C^1}}\|\gamma_+(u_h - u - u')\|_{\mathcal{Y}}$$

$$\leq \frac{\lambda}{\|h_\nu\|_{C^1}}\left(\|\gamma_+(f_h - f - H)\|_{\mathcal{Y}} + \|\gamma_+ L^{-1}S\|\,\|(f_h - f - H)\|_{L^1}\right)$$

$$\to 0 \quad \text{as } h \to 0,$$

where $u_h = \lambda(I + L^{-1}S)f_h$, $u = \lambda(I + L^{-1}S)f$ and $u' = \lambda(I + L^{-1}S)H$. $\quad\square$

Remark 6.16. The domain derivative of F can formally be interpreted as the trace of the 'solution' u' of the transmission boundary value problem

$$\omega \cdot \nabla u' + \sigma_t u' - Su' = \lambda h_\nu \delta|_{\partial\Gamma} \quad \text{in } X \times \Omega \,,$$
$$u' = 0 \quad \text{on } \partial_-(X \times \Omega) \,,$$
(6.26)

as expected from the formal derivative (6.4) and from the derivative in the DA-based framework (4.11). This representation is verified recalling Remark 6.5, where the function H is formally seen as 'solution' of problem (6.26) without scattering and $\lambda = 1$; the solution of the transport equation (6.26) with scattering is then obtained by applying $\lambda(I - \mathcal{K})^{-1} = \lambda(I + L^{-1}S)$ to the function H. Though this observation is only a formal one, we think it is a handy characterization. Therefore, we use it in the following.

Before we finish this section, let us discuss possible generalizations of this approach to more general domains.

Remark 6.17.

(a) The line of argument presented above might be extended to more general domains. A natural choice are convex domains that are diffeomorphic to a ball. The convexity property ensures that there are at most two intersection points of the boundary $\partial\Gamma$ with the line $\{x - t\omega : t \in \mathbb{R}\}$ as in the ball-shaped case. The diffeomorphism allows to map the convex domain back to the ball, which we have considered above. Lines are transformed into curves, whose length can be approximated by the norm of the diffeomorphism. Thus, some of the above results can be generalized.

However, the not yet solved main issue is to handle the integrals of the function $\psi/(\omega \cdot \nu)$. In our proofs we have fundamentally used the fact that Γ is a ball and that the singularity in the integral is the angle between the intersection point $p_i/R = \nu$ and the direction ω. It is still open how to transfer these results to more general domains.[6]

(b) Though we have only developed the domain derivative for balls in the L^1 setting and even showed that it is not possible in L^2, we will see in the upcoming chapter that from a numerically point of view more general domains and the L^2 framework are also feasible.

---

[6]As one might think the restriction to conformal mappings is a remedy to this challenge, we note that it is not, at least in case $d = 3$. In three dimensions all conformal maps are Möbius transformations mapping generalized spheres onto generalized spheres, cf. [**Bea95**, Theorem 15.2] together with [**DFN84**, Theorem 3.2.1].

6.3. Consequences for the Minimization Problem

Knowing the domain derivative of the RTE-based forward operator, at least for ball-shaped sources, we examine the implications to the minimization problem 2.13. First, we calculate the one-sided Hadamard directional derivative of the functional J_α with respect to the geometric variable as well as the intensity variable. Second, we specify the approximate variational principle, Theorem 3.9, further. In comparison to the observations on the DA-based problem in Section 4.2, the results are less significant, since they only hold about balls, where differentiability holds, and only directional derivatives are involved, due to the L^1 norm. Nevertheless, they are important properties and can directly be generalized to domains where F is domain differentiable.

6.3.1. The Directional Derivative of the Minimization Functional J_α.
Before we start with the actual calculation, we have to introduce in which sense we understand the directional derivative. Given a Banach space $\mathcal{X}$ and a functional $\Psi\colon \mathcal{X} \to \mathbb{R}$, we say that Ψ is (one-sided) Hadamard directionally differentiable about $f \in \mathcal{X}$ if for every $h \in \mathcal{X}$ the limit

$$\lim_{\substack{k \to h \\ t \to 0+}} \frac{\Psi(f + tk) - \Psi(f)}{t}$$

exists. In this case, the limit is called (one-sided) Hadamard directional derivative and denoted by $\Psi'(f; h)$. We use this definition rather than the usual (one-sided) Gâteaux directional derivative, since we apply the chain rule later, which does not hold for (one-sided) Gâteaux directionally differentiable functionals in general. For more details on the different notions of directional derivatives we refer to [**Sha90**]. As we do not consider two-sided directional derivatives in this section and as it is also standard in the literature, see e.g. [**IK08, Sha90**], we omit the adjective one-sided subsequently.

The aim of this paragraph is to derive the Hadamard directional derivative of the functional J_α, given by

$$J_\alpha(\lambda, G) = \|F(\lambda, G) - g\|_{\mathcal{Y}} + \alpha \mathrm{Per}(G),$$

with respect to both the intensity and geometric variable. The operator F, defined in (6.3), is linear in the intensity variable. Thus, we have

$$\partial_\lambda F(\lambda, G)k = \sum_{i=1}^{I} k_i A \chi_{G_i}.$$

The domain derivative of $F(\lambda, \cdot)$ about balls is known from Theorem 6.15. Moreover, we recall from Lemma 3.7 that the domain derivative of the penalty term about a smooth domain G is given by

$$\partial_{G_i}\mathrm{Per}(G)h = \int_{\partial G_i} \mathrm{H}_{\partial G_i} h_\nu \, \mathrm{d}\mu$$

with $\mathrm{H}_{\partial G_i}$ being the additive curvature of ∂G_i.

So let us turn to the open point, the calculation of the Hadamard directional derivative of the $\mathcal{Y}$ norm, i.e., the weighted L^1 norm on $\partial_+(X \times \Omega)$. For $f \in \mathcal{Y}$ we define

$$\Psi(f) = \|f\|_{\mathcal{Y}} = \int_\Omega \int_{X_{\omega,+}} |f(y,\omega)| |\omega \cdot \nu(y)| \, \mathrm{d}\mu(y) \, \mathrm{d}\omega \, .$$

By straightforward computations, we observe that

$$\Psi'(f;h) = \int_\Omega \int_{X_{\omega,+}} \mathrm{sgn}\big(f(y,\omega)\big)h(y,\omega)|\omega \cdot \nu(y)| \, \mathrm{d}\mu(y) \, \mathrm{d}\omega \qquad (6.27)$$

$$+ \int_\Omega \int_{X_{\omega,+}} \big(1 - \chi_{\mathrm{supp}\,f}(y,\omega)\big)|h(y,\omega)| |\omega \cdot \nu(y)| \, \mathrm{d}\mu(y) \, \mathrm{d}\omega$$

for $h \in \mathcal{Y}$, where sgn is the sign function

$$\mathrm{sgn}(t) = \begin{cases} 1, & \text{if } t > 0, \\ 0, & \text{if } t = 0, \\ -1, & \text{if } t < 0. \end{cases}$$

Having the Hadamard directional derivative of $\|\cdot\|_{\mathcal{Y}}$ as well as the derivatives of F and Per at hand, an application of the chain rule, see [**DZ11**, Theorem 2.5 in Chapter 9] for instance, yields the following result:

Theorem 6.18 (Directional Derivative of J_α in RTE-based BLT). *Let* $(\lambda, G) \in \Lambda \times \mathcal{G}$ *be such that each component* G_i *is a ball. Then, the functional* J_α *is Hadamard directionally differentiable and for* $k \in \mathbb{R}^I$ *and* $h \in \prod_{i=1}^I C_0^1(X_i, \mathbb{R}^d)$ *holds*

$$J_\alpha\big((\lambda, G); (k, h)\big)$$

$$= \sum_{i=1}^I \left[\Psi'\big(\gamma_+ u - g; k_i \gamma_+ v_i\big) + \Psi'\big(\gamma_+ u - g; \gamma_+ u_i'\big) + \alpha \int_{\partial G_i} \mathrm{H}_{\partial G_i} h_{i,\nu} \, \mathrm{d}\mu \right].$$

Herein, $\gamma_+ u = A \sum_{i=1}^I \lambda_i \chi_{G_i}$, $\gamma_+ v_i = A\chi_{G_i}$ *and* Ψ' *is given in* (6.27). *Moreover,* u_i' *is the solution of the transmission boundary value problem* (6.26) *with* λ, Γ *and* h_ν *replaced by* λ_i, G_i *and* $h_{i,\nu}$, *respectively.*

6.3.2. The Approximate Variational Principle Revisited. In Section 3.2.2 we derived an approximate variational principle, which we specify here. We show that under certain conditions on the minimizer the first-order optimality condition for directional differentiable functionals is approximately satisfied. Since the differentiability of the forward operator F and, thus, of the functional J_α is verified for the small class of ball-shaped sources only, the assumptions are quite restrictive. However, the results can be generalized in a straightforward manner as soon as the domain differentiability of F holds for a broader class. Additionally, we note that, in contrast to the DA-framework in Section 4.2, we do not treat the star-shaped domains separately, since we are only considering ball-shaped sources.[7]

In the derivation of the particular approximate variational principle we cannot directly rely on the general result, Theorem 3.9, since there we assume to have perturbations of G in a subspace of $\prod C_0^2(X_i, \mathbb{R}^d)$. By contrast, we can only consider constant perturbation or perturbation constant in normal direction here, in order to stay in the class of balls. These perturbations do not have compact support.[8] Thus, we have to incorporate a different way to ensure that the perturbed domains remain in the predefined sets X_i. This is simply done by bounding the perturbation.

Let us introduce some notations before we formulate the theorem. Let (λ^*, G^*) be a minimizer of J_α. Further, let $\varepsilon > 0$ and $(\lambda^\varepsilon, G^\varepsilon)$ be such that

$$J_\alpha(\lambda^\varepsilon, G^\varepsilon) \le J_\alpha(\lambda^*, G^*) + \varepsilon \quad \text{and} \quad G_i^\varepsilon = B_{\rho_i}(x_i), \quad i = 1, \dots, I. \quad (6.28)$$

Then, we denote by $\mathcal{V}_i$ the space of admissible perturbations of G_i^ε given by

$$\mathcal{V}_i = \{ r\phi_i + m : r \in \mathbb{R}, m \in \mathbb{R}^d \}, \quad (6.29)$$

where $\phi_i(x) = (x - x_i)/\rho_i$. The perturbations in $\mathcal{V}_i$ are just dilations and translations of G_i, since for $v = r\phi_i + m$ we have $(G_i^\varepsilon)_v = (\mathrm{id} + v)(G_i^\varepsilon) = B_{\rho_i + r}(x_i + m)$. The space $\mathcal{V}_i$ is endowed with the norm

$$\|v\|_{\mathcal{V}_i} = \|v\|_\infty,$$

---

[7]If required, the results in the star-shaped framework are obtained combining the findings in this paragraph with the ones in Section 4.2.3.

[8]By multiplying the constant perturbation with a compactly supported, smooth function one can circumvent this. However, the C^2 norm of this function differs from the absolute value of the constant function in this case, which is not desired.

where $\|\cdot\|_\infty$ is the supremum norm over $G_i^\varepsilon = B_{\rho_i}(x_i)$. Furthermore, we set

$$\mathcal{V} = \prod_{i=1}^{I} \mathcal{V}_i\,.$$

Having these definitions at hand, we can state the specific approximate variational principle: If there exists a ball-shaped source having a J_α-value close to the minimum, then we find another ball-shaped source such that the J_α-value is closer to the minimum and the Hadamard directional derivative about this point in any admissible direction is almost non-negative. Latter means in other words that the first-order optimality condition for directionally differentiable functions is approximately satisfied in this point. The proof is a modification of a consequence of Ekeland's ε-variational principle for directional differentiable functions presented in [**AE84**, Theorem 7.3.6].

Theorem 6.19. *Let (λ^*, G^*) be a minimizer of J_α. Further, let $\varepsilon > 0$ and $(\lambda^\varepsilon, G^\varepsilon)$ be such that (6.28) is satisfied. Moreover, we assume that λ^ε is an inner point of Λ and that*

$$C = \min_{i=1,\ldots,I} \operatorname{dist}(G_i^\varepsilon, \partial X_i) > 0\,.$$

Then for every $\gamma \in]0, \frac{1}{2C}[$ sufficiently small there exist a vector field $v \in \mathcal{V}$ and an intensity $\kappa^\varepsilon \in \Lambda$ with

$$\|(\kappa^\varepsilon - \lambda^\varepsilon, v)\|_{\mathbb{R}^I \times \mathcal{V}} \le \gamma \qquad (6.30)$$

such that the perturbed domain $G_v^\varepsilon = (\operatorname{id} + v)(G^\varepsilon)$ and the intensity κ^ε satisfy

$$J_\alpha(\kappa^\varepsilon, G_v^\varepsilon) \le J_\alpha(\lambda^\varepsilon, G^\varepsilon)\,, \qquad (6.31)$$

$$J_\alpha(\kappa^\varepsilon, G_v^\varepsilon) - \frac{\varepsilon}{\gamma}\|(k,h)\|_{\mathbb{R}^I \times \mathcal{V}} < J_\alpha(\kappa^\varepsilon + k, G_{v+h}^\varepsilon) \qquad (6.32)$$

for all $\kappa^\varepsilon + k \in \Lambda \setminus \{\kappa^\varepsilon\}$ and $v + h \in \mathcal{V} \setminus \{v\}$ with $\|v + h\|_\mathcal{V} \le \frac{1}{2C}$.
In particular,

$$J_\alpha'\big((\kappa^\varepsilon, G_v^\varepsilon); (k, \tilde{h})\big) \ge -\frac{\varepsilon}{\gamma}\|(k, \tilde{h})\|_{\mathbb{R}^I \times C^1} \qquad (6.33)$$

holds for all $(k, \tilde{h}) \in \Lambda \times \widetilde{\mathcal{V}}$. Herein, $\widetilde{\mathcal{V}}$ is defined as in (6.29) but with x_i and ρ_i replaced by y_i and R_i, respectively, where $(G_i^\varepsilon)_{v_i} = B_{R_i}(y_i)$.

PROOF. Let $\mathcal{B}_{\frac{1}{2C}} = \{v \in \mathcal{V}: \|v\|_\mathcal{V} \le \frac{1}{2C}\}$. We consider the functional $\Phi\colon \Lambda \times \mathcal{B}_{\frac{1}{2C}} \to \mathbb{R}$ with $\Phi(\lambda, w) = J_\alpha(\lambda, G_w^\varepsilon)$. Obviously, Φ is continuous in the intensity variable λ. The continuity of J_α in the geometric variable is developed in Section 3.2.2, thus Φ is also continuous in the variable w. The existence of a pair (κ^ε, v) satisfying the three estimates (6.30), (6.31) and (6.32) is an immediate consequence of Ekeland's ε-variational principle, see e.g. [**AE84**, Theorem 5.3.1].

It remains to show the inequality (6.33). We derive it from estimate (6.32) together with the Hadamard directional differentiability of J_α. Let $(k, h) \in \mathbb{R}^I \times \mathcal{V} \setminus \{(0,0)\}$ and $t > 0$. In view of (6.32), we have

$$-\frac{\varepsilon}{\gamma}\|(tk, th)\|_{\mathbb{R}^I \times \mathcal{V}} < J_\alpha(\kappa^\varepsilon + tk, G^\varepsilon_{v+th}) - J_\alpha(\kappa^\varepsilon, G^\varepsilon_v).$$

With the definition $\widetilde{h} = h \circ (\mathrm{id} + v)^{-1}$ and the observation $G^\varepsilon_{v+th} = (G^\varepsilon_v)_{\widetilde{th}}$ follows that

$$-\frac{\varepsilon}{\gamma}\|(tk, th)\|_{\mathbb{R}^I \times \mathcal{V}} < J_\alpha\left(\kappa^\varepsilon + tk, (G^\varepsilon_v)_{\widetilde{th}}\right) - J_\alpha(\kappa^\varepsilon, G^\varepsilon_v).$$

Letting $t \to 0$ and taking the Hadamard directional differentiability of J_α into account[9], cf. Theorem 6.18, we obtain

$$-\frac{\varepsilon}{\gamma}\|(k, h)\|_{\mathbb{R}^I \times \mathcal{V}} \leq J'_\alpha\left((\kappa^\varepsilon, G^\varepsilon_v); (k, \widetilde{h})\right).$$

Moreover, we observe that every element $\widetilde{w} \in \widetilde{\mathcal{V}}$ can be written in the form $w \circ (\mathrm{id} + v)^{-1}$ with $w \in \mathcal{V}$ and vice versa. Using this fact and the identity

$$\|\widetilde{h}\|_{\widetilde{\mathcal{V}}} = \|h\|_{\mathcal{V}},$$

we finally obtain that (6.33) holds for all $(k, \widetilde{h}) \in \Lambda \times \widetilde{\mathcal{V}}$. $\square$

---

[9]Herein, we also use the fact that the domain derivative only depends on the normal component of the perturbation on the boundary of G. Therefore, it does not matter that the elements of $\mathcal{V}$ do not have compact support in X_i.

CHAPTER 7

Numerical Experiments for RTE-based Bioluminescence Tomography

In this chapter we complement the study of the RTE-based BLT problem by looking at it from a numerical point of view. Although we have developed the domain differentiability of the forward operator only for ball-shaped sources, we, somehow heuristically, consider general star-shaped domains here. In addition, we work in the L^2 framework despite Remark 6.7, which tells us that this setting does not work theoretically. Latter relaxation simplifies the calculation of the gradient of J_α in Section 7.1.1. Moreover, it allows us to use the discrete-ordinate discontinuous Galerkin method developed in [**HHE10**] to solve the radiative transfer equation in Section 7.2. We see in the upcoming numerical experiments that neither the lack of theory nor the mismatched space do cause any problems in the numerics.

This chapter is organized as Chapter 5. In Section 7.1 we recall the projected gradient method and split approach from Section 5.1 for the sake of completeness. In addition, we calculate the ingredients for these algorithms, namely the gradient and projection in the transport framework. Several numerical experiments in three dimensions are presented in Section 7.2. We note that the intention of this chapter is to illustrate the applicability of the geometric regularization approach in RTE-based BLT, rather than to give the most sophisticated implementation and most complete discussion of the proposed scheme.

7.1. Numerical Schemes

Before we restate the descent methods to solve the minimization problem 2.13 for star-shaped domains, we calculate the gradient of J_α and recall the projections needed in the algorithms. In order to simplify the implementation, we entirely work in the Hilbert space setting. The parameterizations of the star-shaped domains are assumed to lie in a Hilbert space $\mathcal{U}$ that is a dense subspace of $C^2(S^{d-1})^I$. The image space is set to

$$\mathcal{Y}_2 = L^2\big(\partial_+(X \times \Omega), |\omega \cdot \nu| \, \mathrm{d}\omega \, \mathrm{d}\mu\big). \tag{7.1}$$

We point out that all following calculations have to be understood in a formal way, so that we circumvent any issues due to the L^2 framework. The operators A and F as well as the functional J_α are adapted according to the choice of $\mathcal{U}$ and $\mathcal{Y}_2$. As in Section 5.1, we denote by $\mathcal{R}_{\mathrm{ad}} \subset (\mathcal{U} \times \mathbb{R}^{dI}) \cap \mathcal{R}$ the set of admissible star-shaped domains, which is assumed to be closed and convex. In addition, we define the closed and convex set $\mathcal{C} = \Lambda \times \mathcal{R}_{\mathrm{ad}}$ and $\Pi_\mathcal{C}$ as the convex projection onto $\mathcal{C}$.

Having introduced the framework and notation, the minimization problem under consideration in this numerical chapter is:

$$\text{Minimize } J_\alpha(\lambda, r, m) = \frac{1}{2}\big\|F(\lambda, r, m) - g\big\|_{\mathcal{Y}_2}^2 + \alpha \mathrm{Per}(r) \text{ over } \mathcal{C}.$$

7.1.1. Gradient and Projection. Before we start with the actual discussion, we point out that the results in this paragraph are similar to the ones in Section 5.1.1. Roughly speaking, the only modifications are that we replace the diffusion approximation by the radiative transfer equation and that we consider $d = 3$ instead of $d = 2$ in the dimension specific calculations. However, we present the entire argument for the sake of completeness.

We recall that the gradient of J_α has to satisfy

$$\langle \mathrm{grad}\, J_\alpha(\lambda, r, m), (h_\lambda, h_r, h_m)\rangle_{\mathbb{R}^I \times \mathcal{U} \times \mathbb{R}^{dI}} = J_\alpha'(\lambda, r, m)(h_\lambda, h_r, h_m).$$

The occurring (formal) derivative J_α' is easily obtained combining the representation (6.4) of the formal derivative of F with the derivative of J_α in the DA-framework, compare Theorem 4.2. Consequently,

$$\langle \operatorname{grad} J_\alpha(\lambda, r, m), (h_\lambda, h_r, h_m) \rangle_{\mathbb{R}^I \times \mathcal{U} \times \mathbb{R}^{dI}}$$
$$= \langle F(\lambda, r, m) - g, \partial_\lambda F(\lambda, r, m) h_\lambda + \partial_r F(\lambda, r, m) h_r + \partial_m F(\lambda, r, m) h_m \rangle_{\mathcal{Y}_2}$$
$$+ \alpha \partial_r \operatorname{Per}(r) h_r$$
$$= \sum_{i=1}^I \Big(\langle \gamma_+ u - g, h_{\lambda,i} \gamma_+ v_i + \gamma_+ u'_{r,i} + \gamma_+ u'_{m,i} \rangle_{\mathcal{Y}_2}$$
$$+ \alpha \int_{\partial G_i} \mathrm{H}_{\partial G_i} h_{r,i} \cdot \nu \, d\mu \Big).$$

Herein, $\gamma_+ u = A \sum_{i=1}^I \lambda_i \chi_{G_i}$ and $\gamma_+ v_i = A \chi_{G_i}$. Moreover, the terms $u'_{r,i}$ and $u_{m,i}$ are the solutions of the transmission boundary value problem (6.26) with h replaced by $h_{r,i}$ and $h_{m,i}$, respectively, as well as Γ replaced by G_i and λ by λ_i.

Since we select $\mathcal{U}$ to be a Sobolev space H^s on the unit sphere S^{d-1} later, we are particularly interested in the H^s gradient. As mentioned in Section 5.1, the H^s gradient can be calculated from the L^2 gradient by multiplying the Fourier coefficients associated with spherical harmonics of degree j by $(1 + j^2)^{-s}$ if $d = 2$ and by $(j + 1/2)^{-2s}$ if $d = 3$. See [Kre89] and [FGS98], respectively, for more details. Thus, we start with the computation of the L^2 gradient.

The components of the L^2 gradient[1] have to satisfy

$$\begin{aligned}
\big(\operatorname{grad} J_\alpha(\lambda, r, m)\big)_{\lambda_i} &= \langle F(\lambda, r, m) - g, A\chi_{G_i} \rangle_{\mathcal{Y}}, \\
\big(\operatorname{grad} J_\alpha(\lambda, r, m)\big)_{r_i} &= \partial_{r_i} F(\lambda, r, m)^* \big(F(\lambda, r, m) - g\big) \\
&\quad + \alpha \mathrm{H}_{\partial G_i} (\Phi_1 \cdot \nu) \sqrt{\operatorname{gr} \Phi'_{r_i}}, \\
\big(\operatorname{grad} J_\alpha(\lambda, r, m)\big)_{m_i} &= \partial_{m_i} F(\lambda, r, m)^* \big(F(\lambda, r, m) - g\big),
\end{aligned} \tag{7.2}$$

where Φ_1 is the parameterization of the unit sphere and $\operatorname{gr} \Phi'_\rho$ is the Gramian determinant of the derivative of the parameterization Φ_ρ of $\partial\Gamma$. We specify the components of the L^2 gradient in three dimension, since this is the case we consider in all numerical experiments of the next section. The two-dimensional case can be treated similar to Section 5.1.

In case $d = 3$, the second equation in (7.2) can be rewritten as

$$\big(\operatorname{grad} J_\alpha(\lambda, r, m)\big)_{r_i} = \partial_{r_i} F(\lambda, r, m)^* \big(F(\lambda, r, m) - g\big) + \alpha \mathrm{H}_{\partial G_i} r_i^2, \tag{7.3}$$

where the L^2 adjoint of $\partial_{r_i} F(\lambda, r, m)$ is derived as follows: For $\psi \in \mathcal{Y}_2$ let $w \in W^2(X \times \Omega) = \{v \in L^2(X \times \Omega) : \omega \cdot \nabla v \in L^2(X \times \Omega)\}$ be the solution

---

[1]We use the same convention for the subscripts as in Section 5.1.1.

of the adjoint boundary value problem

$$-\omega \cdot \nabla w + \sigma_t w - S w = 0 \quad \text{in } X \times \Omega \,,$$
$$w = \psi \quad \text{on } \partial_+ (X \times \Omega) \,. \tag{7.4}$$

For an existence and uniqueness result we refer to [**CZ67, DL00b**]. Using the integration by parts formula

$$\int_\Omega \int_X (\omega \cdot \nabla v) w + v(\omega \cdot \nabla w) \, \mathrm{d}x \, \mathrm{d}\omega = \int_\Omega \int_{\partial X} v w \, (\omega \cdot \nu) \, \mathrm{d}\mu \, \mathrm{d}\omega \,,$$

we obtain

$$
\begin{aligned}
\langle \partial_{r_i} F(\lambda, r, m) h_{r,i}, \psi \rangle_{\mathcal{Y}_2} &= \int_\Omega \int_{\partial X} u'_{r,i} w \, (\omega \cdot \nu) \, \mathrm{d}\mu \, \mathrm{d}\omega \\
&= \int_\Omega \int_X (\omega \cdot \nabla u'_{r,i}) w + u'_{r,i} (\omega \cdot \nabla w) \, \mathrm{d}x \, \mathrm{d}\omega \\
&= \lambda_i \int_\Omega \int_{\partial G_i} w \, (h_{r,i} \cdot \nu) \circ \Phi_{r_i}^{-1} \, \mathrm{d}\mu \, \mathrm{d}\omega \\
&= \int_{S^2} \lambda_i h_{r,i} r_i^2 w \circ \Phi_{r_i} \, \mathrm{d}\mu \\
&= \langle h_{r,i}, \partial_{r_i} F(\lambda, r, m)^* \psi \rangle_{L^2} \,.
\end{aligned}
$$

Thus, the L^2 adjoint admits the representation

$$\partial_{r_i} F(\lambda, r, m)^* \psi = \lambda_i r_i^2 \int_\Omega w|_{\partial G_i} \big(\Phi_{r_i}(\,\cdot\,), \omega \big) \, \mathrm{d}\omega \,. \tag{7.5}$$

The adjoint of $\partial_{m_i} F(\lambda, m, r)$, occurring in the last equation of (7.2), is derived in a similar way. It has the form

$$\partial_{m_i} F(\lambda, r, m)^* \psi = \lambda_i \int_\Omega \int_{\partial G_i} w \nu \, \mathrm{d}\mu \, \mathrm{d}\omega \,, \tag{7.6}$$

where w is still the solution of the adjoint boundary value problem (7.4).

For the sake of completeness, we recall the projection operator in λ onto the interval $\Lambda = \prod [\underline{\lambda}_i, \overline{\lambda}_i]$ from Section 5.1. It is given by

$$(\Pi_{\mathcal{C}}^\lambda \lambda)_i = \begin{cases} \underline{\lambda}_i \,, & \lambda_i < \underline{\lambda}_i \,, \\ \overline{\lambda}_i \,, & \lambda_i > \overline{\lambda}_i \,, \\ \lambda_i \,, & \text{otherwise} \,. \end{cases}$$

As in the DA-framework, the convex projection in (r, m) onto $\mathcal{R}_{\mathrm{ad}}$ is not implemented, since in the numerical experiments the iterates stay in $\mathcal{R}_{\mathrm{ad}}$ for suitable initial values.

7.1.2. Projected Gradient Method. One of the used optimization schemes is the projected gradient method, which is taken from [**HPUU09**] and described in Algorithm 7.1. The projected Armijo rule is applied to find the step size s_k: The largest $s_k \in \{\frac{1}{2^n} : n \in \mathbb{N}_0\}$ is chosen such that

$$J_\alpha\Big(\Pi_{\mathcal{C}}\big((\lambda^k, r^k, m^k) + s_k(h_\lambda^k, h_r^k, h_m^k)\big)\Big) - J_\alpha(\lambda^k, r^k, m^k)$$

$$\leq -\frac{\gamma}{s_k}\Big\|\Pi_{\mathcal{C}}\big((\lambda^k, r^k, m^k) + s_k(h_\lambda^k, h_r^k, h_m^k)\big) - (\lambda^k, r^k, m^k)\Big\|_{\mathbb{R}^I \times \mathcal{U} \times \mathbb{R}^{dI}}^2$$

with some constant $\gamma \in]0, 1[$.

Algorithm 7.1 Projected Gradient Method

(S0) Choose $(\lambda^0, r^0, m^0) \in \mathcal{C}$.

For $k = 0, 1, 2, \ldots$

(S1) Test for termination.

(S2) Set $(h_\lambda^k, h_r^k, h_m^k) = -\operatorname{grad} J_\alpha(\lambda^k, r^k, m^k)$.

(S3) Choose s_k by a projected step size rule such that

$$J_\alpha\Big(\Pi_{\mathcal{C}}\big((\lambda^k, r^k, m^k) + s_k(h_\lambda^k, h_r^k, h_m^k)\big)\Big) < J_\alpha(\lambda^k, r^k, m^k).$$

(S4) Set $(\lambda^{k+1}, r^{k+1}, m^{k+1}) = \Pi_{\mathcal{C}}\big((\lambda^k, r^k, m^k) + s_k(h_\lambda^k, h_r^k, h_m^k)\big)$.

7.1.3. Split Approach. The other optimization scheme we apply later is the so-called split approach. Inspired by [**RR07**], we split the kth iteration into the following two steps:

$$\lambda^{k+1} = \underset{\lambda \in \Lambda}{\arg\min}\, J_\alpha(\lambda, r^k, m^k),$$

$$(r^{k+1}, m^{k+1}) = \Pi_{\mathcal{R}_{\mathrm{ad}}}\big((r^k, m^k) - s_k(h_r^k, h_m^k)\big)$$

with

$$h_r^k = \big(\operatorname{grad} J_\alpha(\lambda^{k+1}, r^k, m^k)\big)_r \quad \text{and} \quad h_m^k = \big(\operatorname{grad} J_\alpha(\lambda^{k+1}, r^k, m^k)\big)_m.$$

The step size s_k is chosen by the projected Armijo rule as above. This leads to Algorithm 7.2.

For a detailed discussion of the optimization problem in step (S2) we refer to Section 5.1.3.

Algorithm 7.2 Split Approach

   (S0) Choose $(\lambda^0, r^0, m^0) \in \mathcal{C}$.

For $k = 0, 1, 2, \ldots$

   (S1) Test for termination.

   (S2) Calculate $\lambda^{k+1} = \arg\min_{\lambda \in \Lambda} J_\alpha(\lambda, r^k, m^k)$.

   (S3) Set $(h_r^k, h_m^k) = -\left(\text{grad}\, J_\alpha(\lambda^{k+1}, r^k, m^k)\right)_{(r,m)}$.

   (S4) Choose s_k by a projected step size rule such that

$$J_\alpha\left(\lambda^{k+1}, \Pi_{\mathcal{R}_{\text{ad}}}\left((r^k, m^k) + s_k(h_r^k, h_m^k)\right)\right) < J_\alpha(\lambda^{k+1}, r^k, m^k).$$

   (S5) Set $(r^{k+1}, m^{k+1}) = \Pi_{\mathcal{R}_{\text{ad}}}\left((r^k, m^k) + s_k(h_r^k, h_m^k)\right)$.

7.2. Numerical Examples

After the discussion of the used optimization methods and the required quantities in these algorithms, let us turn to the numerical experiments. We start explaining the implementation. Then, reconstructions of different sources are presented. For the sake of simplicity, we restrict ourselves to the situation where the source term consists of only one characteristic function: $q = \lambda \chi_G$. The more general situation of I characteristic functions poses no principal problems, compare Section 5.2.5 for the reconstruction of two sources in the DA-framework.

7.2.1. Implementation. All following numerical experiments are performed in three dimensions. To solve the occurring boundary value problems the program RTEPACK written by Joseph Eichholz is used. It implements the discrete-ordinate discontinuous Galerkin (DODG) method described in [**HHE10, Eic11**] for solving the radiative transfer equation. See [**Eic13**] for details on RTEPACK. We give more information on the used discretization of the scattering operator S later. The spatial domain X is triangulated into tetrahedral elements with mesh size h and the space of local linear elements is chosen.

Let (r, m) be a parameterization of the searched-for domain G. We approximate the function r by a spherical polynomial[2] r_M of degree less than M:

$$r(\theta) \approx r_M(\theta) = \sum_{n=0}^{M} \sum_{l=-n}^{n} \gamma_{n,l} Y_{n,l}(\theta) \tag{7.7}$$

---

[2]In two dimensions trigonometric polynomial can be used, see Chapter 5.

for $\theta \in S^2$. Herein, $Y_{n,l}$ is the spherical harmonic of degree n and order l, see Appendix A.2 for the definition and properties, and the coefficients $\gamma_{n,l}$ are given by

$$\gamma_{n,l} = \langle r, Y_{n,l} \rangle_{L^2} = \int_{S^2} r(\theta) Y_{n,l}(\theta) \, d\theta. \tag{7.8}$$

Now, the numerical experiments are performed on the vector of Fourier coefficients

$$(\gamma_{0,0}, \gamma_{1,0}, \gamma_{1,-1}, \gamma_{1,1}, \ldots, \gamma_{M,M})$$

rather than on the function r_M itself.

In view of this discretization of r, a matched discretization of the following terms is needed:

1. the source term q, i.e., the scaled characteristic function $\lambda \chi_G$,
2. the L^2 adjoint of $\partial_r F(\lambda, r, m)$, see (7.5), and
3. the gradient of the perimeter, see (3.5).

As a reminder, the items No. 2 and No. 3 occur in the second component of the L^2 gradient $(\mathrm{grad}\, J_\alpha(\lambda, r, m))_r$ given in (7.3).

Before we describe the treatment of the above quantities, we note that they are handled in an analogous manner as the corresponding quantities in the DA-framework in Section 5.2. In principle, the only modifications are the substitution of the radiative transfer equation for the diffusion approximation and the change from trigonometric polynomials to spherical polynomials. The detailed handling of these terms is explained in the following:

1. Let G_M be the star-shaped domain parameterized by (r_M, m). The discretized source function q_h is obtained by interpolation of the scaled characteristic function of G_M in the finite element space. Then, the DODG method implemented in RTEPACK is applied to evaluate the linear forward operator A.
2. To calculate the L^2 adjoint of $\partial_r F(\lambda, r, m)$, the numerical solution of the adjoint boundary value problem (7.4), obtained by the DODG method, is evaluated at the intersection points of the triangulation of X and the boundary ∂G_M. At these spatial points the integral in the angular variable over the unit sphere Ω is computed by the quadrature rule also used in the discrete-ordinate step of the DODG method, i.e., the quadrature rule to approximate the scattering operator S. The resulting local linear function in the spatial variable is multiplied by λr_M^2 and its first $(M+1)^2$ Fourier coefficients (7.8) are approximated by the composite method, see [AH12, Section 5.2+5.4], where the nodes agree with the intersection points. We point out that, due to

the discontinuity of the numerical solution, each intersection point has to be considered several times and in dependence on the tetrahedron it lies in.

3. For the computation of the Fourier coefficients (7.8) of the gradient of the perimeter term, which is given by the product $H_{\partial G_M} r_M^2$, we apply the product Gaußian quadrature formula, cf. [**AH12**, Section 5.1]. Since both functions $H_{\partial G_M}$ and r_M are explicitly known on S^2, it is possible to use this more accurate quadrature rule.

The discretized version of the adjoint operator $\partial_m F(\lambda, r, m)^*$, given in (7.6), is calculated similarly to No. 2 above: The numerical solution of the adjoint boundary value problem (7.4) is first evaluated at the intersection points of the spatial FE mesh and the boundary of G_M. At these points, the solution is integrated in the angular variable over the unit sphere Ω, applying the quadrature rule of the discrete-ordinate method. Then, the resulting local linear function is multiplied by λ times the unit normal ν. In the last step, the integral of the product over ∂G_M is computed by the composite method, where the nodes are given by the intersection points.

As mentioned in the previous section, we do not implement the projection onto $\mathcal{R}_{\mathrm{ad}}$, since for suitable initial values the iterates stay in this set. Only the projection of λ onto Λ is used

For the Hilbert space $\mathcal{U}$ we choose the Sobolev space $H^4(S^2)$, which is a subspace of $C^2(S^2)$, see [**FGS98**, Lemma 5.2.3] for instance. In this setting, the theory developed in the previous chapters is applicable. However, we also consider the L^2 setting, which is not covered by the theory, since we have observed in the DA-framework in Section 5.2 that the $H^3(0, 2\pi)$ gradient has an intrinsic smoothing property leading to almost ball-shaped sources.

The major contributors to the computational costs are the same three components of the reconstruction procedure as in the DA-framework: the solutions of the direct and the adjoint boundary value problems (2.20) and (7.4) as well as the determination of the intersection points of the spatial FE mesh and the boundary of G_M, cf. No. 2 above. The direct problem has to be solved repeatedly to determine the step size s_k in both Algorithms 7.1 and 7.2 by the Armijo rule. The other two costly operations are performed only once per iteration step. However, due to the dependence on both the spatial and angular variable, the costs of solving the radiative transfer equation are significantly higher than of solving the diffusion equation.

In the choice of the termination criterion we follow again [**Kel99**] and use a combination of a relative and an absolute measure of the gradient.

The gradient iteration is stopped if

$$\left\|(h_\lambda^k, h_r^k, h_m^k)\right\|_{\mathbb{R}\times\mathcal{U}\times\mathbb{R}^d} \leq \tau_a + \tau_r \left\|(h_\lambda^0, h_r^0, h_m^0)\right\|_{\mathbb{R}\times\mathcal{U}\times\mathbb{R}^d}$$

and the split approach if

$$\left\|(h_r^k, h_m^k)\right\|_{\mathbb{R}\times\mathcal{U}} \leq \tau_a + \tau_r \left\|(h_r^0, h_m^0)\right\|_{\mathcal{U}\times\mathbb{R}^d},$$

where the notation of Algorithm 7.1 and 7.2 is used. The relative and absolute tolerances are chosen as $\tau_r = \tau_a = 0.005$ for both numerical schemes. In addition, the reconstruction procedures are terminated after maximal 50 iterations, owing to the long computing time.[3] Further, the parameter γ in the projected Armijo rule is set to $5 \cdot 10^{-5}$ and the step size s is bounded between 2^{-8} and 2^{-1}.

In order to improve the reconstructions, the methods described in Algorithm 7.1 and 7.2 are modified in following three ways:

1. The degree M of the spherical polynomial r_M approximating the function r is selected adaptively. At the beginning of the reconstruction scheme M is set to zero, so that only the radius of the source is determined. After every 5 iterations, M is increased by one until the maximal desired degree $M_{\max}$ is reached. This leads to a rough reconstruction in the early stages, but more details are added during further progress of the iterative schemes.

2. In many experiments we observe that at the beginning of the reconstruction process the gradient of J_α is highly dominated by the component in the intensity variable λ. In the gradient method, this prevents changes in the geometry variables m and r. In order to counteract against this, we normalize each of the components if they are too large. If all components are small, the usual gradient is used. More precisely, we use in the 'gradient method' the search direction

$$\left(\frac{h_\lambda^k}{\max\{|h_\lambda^k|, 1\}}, \frac{h_r^k}{\max\{\|h_r^k\|_{\mathcal{U}}, 1\}}, \frac{h_m^k}{\max\{|h_m^k|, 1\}} \right)$$

instead of the negative gradient $(h_\lambda^k, h_r^k, h_m^k)$ as described in step (S2) of Algorithm 7.1.[4]

---

[3]On the used machine 50 iterations take approximately 5 hours, though parts of the code, like solving the transport equation, run parallel on 12 processors.

[4]We notice that this is actually not a gradient method any more. Nevertheless, we still call it like this, since at least near a stationary point the method coincides with the gradient method. Moreover, we point out that the modified search direction remains to be a descent direction.

3. When using the split approach, we notice in many experiments that the gradient of J_α in the geometric variables r and m is large in the beginning of the reconstruction process. This leads to too large steps, which implies an elimination of the source due to negative parameterization or location outside of the object. To prevent such a behavior, the gradient of J_α in the geometric variables is normalized if its norm is larger than 1.

7.2.2. Phantom. The phantom we use in all our computations in the RTE-framework is a homogeneous cylinder with radius 3 and height 6. The total attenuation coefficient σ_t and the scattering coefficient σ_s are set to 1.1 and 1, respectively. For the scattering kernel η we use the Henyey-Greenstein phase function, cf. [**HG41**], which is defined by

$$\eta(t) = \frac{1 - \beta^2}{4\pi(1 + \beta^2 - 2\beta t)^{3/2}} \quad \text{for } t \in [-1, 1].$$

This function describes light scattering in tissue well [**Klo09**] and is, therefore, widely used as scattering kernel. The parameter $\beta \in \,]-1, 1[$ is called anisotropy factor, as it is a measure for anisotropy in the medium. We choose $\beta = 0.8$ in our experiments.

Let us point out that we are aware that this phantom is not a model for the typical object in bioluminescence tomography. According to [**Arr02**], the absorption coefficient σ_a and the scattering coefficient σ_s typically range from 0.01 to 1 mm^{-1} and from 10 to 20 mm^{-1}, respectively, in tissue.[5] A typical value of the anisotropy factor in tissue is around $\beta = 0.9$. Moreover, the usual object under observation is a mouse, whose diameter and length is a few centimeters. Running numerical experiments with such a phantom requires a fine discretization, especially in the angular variable, in order that a discrete analog to the subcritical condition (2.18) is satisfied, see [**Eic11**] for details. This goes beyond the scope of this work. Once again, we emphasize that the numerical experiments serve as proof of concept and as numerical validation of the theoretical findings from the previous chapters.

7.2.3. Model 1. In the first experiment we want to verify the main result of Section 6.2, the domain differentiability of the RTE-based forward operator about balls, numerically. The searched-for source is ball-shaped with radius 1 and centered at $(1.5, 0.5, 0)$. Its intensity λ is set to 1. We illustrate the source inside the phantom in Figure 7.1. The synthetic data are produced on a spatial mesh with mesh size 0.7 and employing the level

---

[5]We recall the relation $\sigma_t = \sigma_a + \sigma_s$.

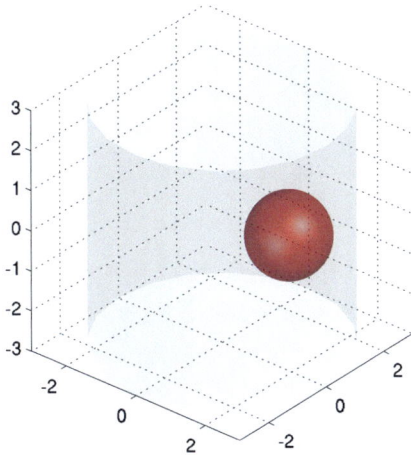

FIGURE 7.1. Sketch of Model 1: searched-for source (red) inside the phantom (gray).

symmetric quadrature S_8, see [**LM84**], for the discretization in the angular variable. Thereby, the right-hand side of the DODG system is assembled with the standard RTEPACK quadrature rule over a tetrahedron, which is a Gauß quadrature of degree 5, using the exact source function q. Though we apply the same discretization of $X \times \Omega$ to solve the inverse problem, the most obvious inverse crime is avoided by a different assembly of the right-hand side in the DODG system.[6] Instead of the exact source q, its projection q_h onto the finite element space is used. The resulting relative discretization error in the data of 7% may be interpreted as 'modeling' error.

Since we want to verify the theory of the previous chapter in this experiment, we assume a ball-shaped source. Consequently, we set the maximal degree M_{max} of the spherical polynomial in (7.7) to 0. For the intensity variable λ we allow a variation of 30%, that is, we choose $\Lambda = [0.7, 1.3]$. The regularization parameter $\alpha = 10^{-9}$ is selected a priori for all our experiments. The iteration is initialized with $\lambda^0 = 0.7$, $m^0 = (0,0,0)$ and $r^0 \equiv 1.5$, which implies an initial relative discrete L^2 error of 150%.

---

[6]We are aware that we still commit an inverse crime, as we use the same numerical method to generate the data and to solve the inverse problem. However, we accept this, in view of the 'modeling' error and the purpose of the numerical experiments.

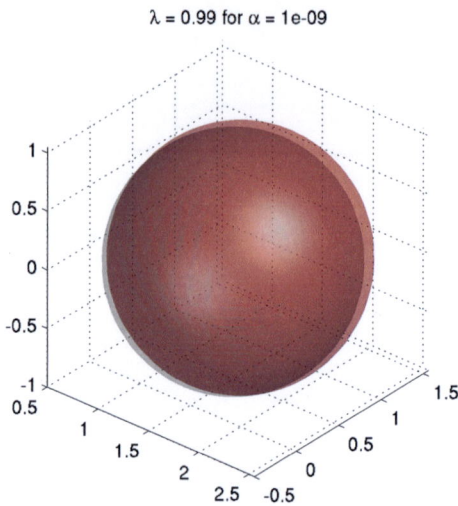

FIGURE 7.2. Reconstruction (red) and original source (gray) after 50 gradient iterations. The relative discrete L^2 error is 1%.

Herein, a discrete L^2 norm of the source function q over the spatial domain X is considered.

After 50 gradient iterations the reconstruction shown in Figure 7.2 is obtained. We observe that the location of the source and the intensity is well reconstructed. The relative discrete L^2 error is reduced to 1%.

7.2.4. Model 2. In the second model we consider a star-shaped source that is not ball-shaped, in order to investigate the applicability of the proposed geometric approach in this more general setting from a numerical point of view. The searched-for source is centered at the point $(1.5, 0.5, 0)$ and its boundary is parameterized by the spherical polynomial

$$r(\theta) = 1 + 0.25\sqrt{\frac{4\pi}{3}}Y_{1,0}(\theta) - 0.15\sqrt{\frac{12\pi}{5}}Y_{2,1}(\theta) \quad \text{for } \theta \in S^2 .$$

The intensity λ equals 1. A sketch of the source inside the phantom is found in Figure 7.3. For the synthetic data generation as well as the solution of the inverse problem the same discretization as in Model 1 is used. This results in a 'modeling' error of 8%.

In all experiments based on Model 2 we set the maximal degree of the spherical polynomial $M_{\max} = 5$ and the admissible interval $\Lambda = [0.7, 1.3]$.

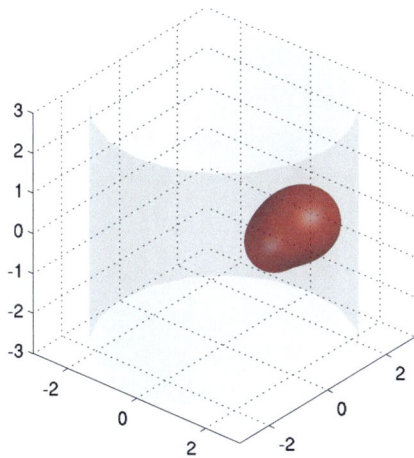

FIGURE 7.3. Sketch of Model 2: searched-for source (red) inside the phantom (gray).

Former selection ensures that the searched-for parameterization lies in the ansatz space, that is, $r = r_M$ in (7.7). Moreover, we choose the initial values $\lambda^0 = 0.7$, $m^0 = (0,0,0)$ and $r^0 \equiv 1.5$ in all experiments of this paragraph, which yields an initial relative discrete L^2 error of 145%.

7.2.4.1. H^4 vs. L^2 setting. In Figure 7.4 the reconstruction after 50 gradient iterations in the H^4 setting is illustrated. As in the diffusion model, we observe that the reconstructed domain resembles a ball because of the inherent smoothing of the H^4 gradient. By comparison, the shape of the source is better reconstructed applying the gradient method in the L^2 setting. This reconstruction is presented in Figure 7.5. The different quality of the reconstructions becomes also apparent in the relative discrete L^2 errors, which read 35% in the H^4 setting and 16% in the L^2 setting.

7.2.4.2. Noisy data. In the experiment presented in Figure 7.6 the synthetic data are corrupted by 30% relative Gaußian noise with respect to a discrete $\mathcal{Y}_2$ norm, cf. (7.1). After 50 split approach iterations the relative discrete L^2 error is reduced to 23%. For comparison, the noise-free reconstruction shown in Figure 7.7 admits a relative discrete L^2 error of 18%. Also the visually noticeable difference in both the shape and intensity of the source is gradual. We conclude that the reconstruction is stable due to the regularizing effects of the perimeter penalty term, the low degree of the spherical polynomial r_M and the upper bound on the

$\lambda = 0.8955$ for $\alpha = 1e-09$

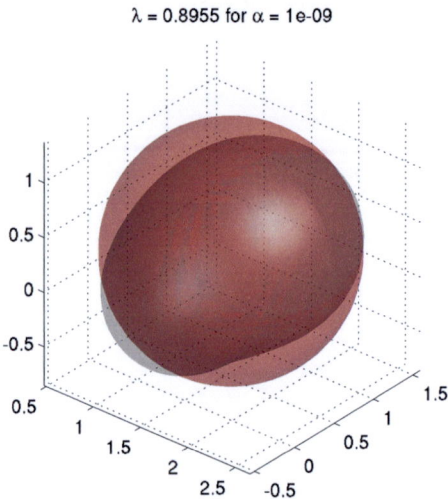

FIGURE 7.4. H^4 setting: Reconstruction (red) and original source (gray) after 50 gradient iterations. The relative discrete L^2 error is 35%.

$\lambda = 0.9493$ for $\alpha = 1e-09$

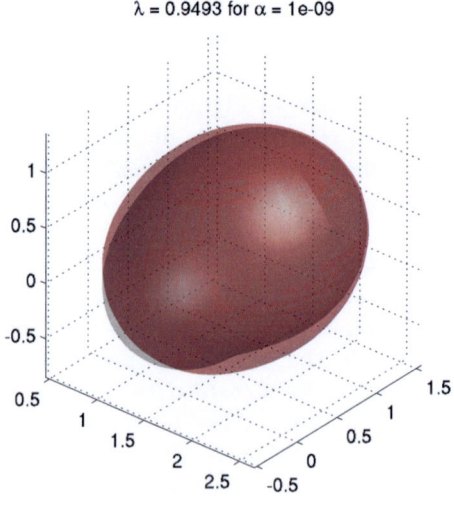

FIGURE 7.5. L^2 setting: Reconstruction (red) and original source (gray) after 50 gradient iterations. The relative discrete L^2 error is 16%.

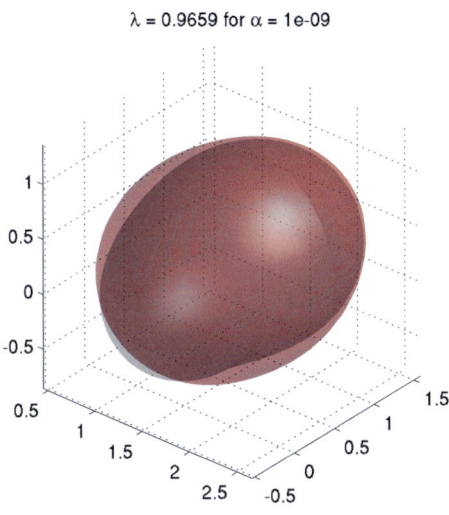

λ = 0.9659 for α = 1e-09

FIGURE 7.6. L^2 setting: Reconstruction (red) and original source (gray) with 30% noise level after 50 split approach iterations. The relative discrete L^2 error is 23%.

number of iterations. We note that in this experiment the latter two have the highest impact on the stabilization, since the regularization parameter α is chosen very small.

7.2.5. Model 3. In the third model the searched-for domain is star-shaped but not explicitly given as an element of the ansatz space. Inspired by [**IK10**], the source is cushion-shaped with center $(1, 0.5, 0)$ and boundary parameterization

$$ r(\theta) = \sqrt{0.8 + 0.5\big(\cos(2\phi) - 1\big)\big(\cos(4\vartheta) - 1\big)} $$

for $\theta = (\cos\phi\sin\vartheta, \sin\phi\sin\vartheta, \cos\vartheta)^T \in S^2$. Its intensity is set to $\lambda = 1$. The location of the source inside the phantom is displayed in Figure 7.8. The synthetic data are produced using the same discretization as in Model 1. For solving the inverse problems we also employ the discretization described above. This results in a 'modeling' error of 7%.

The *a priori* knowledge on the intensity is again implemented by setting $\Lambda = [0.7, 1.3]$. In both experiments based on Model 3 the following

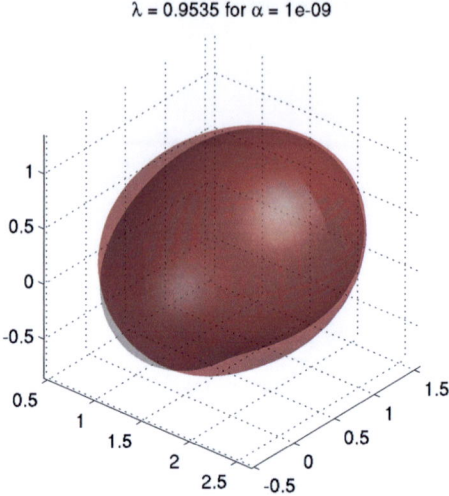

FIGURE 7.7. L^2 setting: Reconstruction (red) and original source (gray) after 50 split approach iterations. The relative discrete L^2 error is 18%.

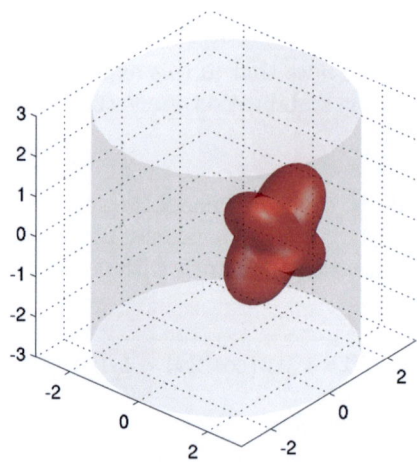

FIGURE 7.8. Sketch of Model 3: searched-for source (red) inside the phantom (gray).

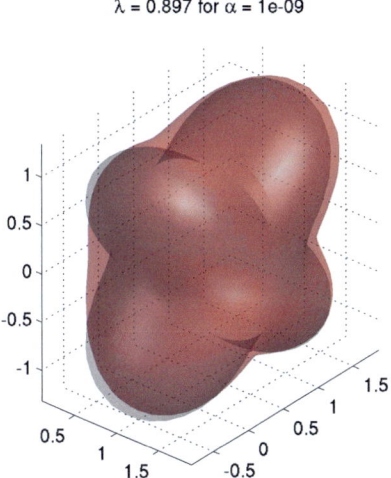

λ = 0.897 for α = 1e-09

FIGURE 7.9. L^2 setting, $M_{max} = 5$: Reconstruction (red) and original source (gray) after 50 gradient iterations. The relative discrete L^2 error is 26%.

initial values are chosen: $\lambda^0 = 0.7$, $m^0 = (0,0,0)$ and $r^0 \equiv 1.5$. Thus, the initial relative discrete L^2 error is 115%.

For maximal degree $M_{max} = 5$ and $M_{max} = 8$, the reconstructions after 50 gradient iterations are shown in Figure 7.9 and 7.10, respectively. We observe that the cushion is quite well reconstructed in both cases. However, the reconstruction of the intensity as well as the shape is better for the higher degree, $M_{max} = 8$. In this case, the relative discrete L^2 error reduces to 18%, which is about the same size as the errors in Model 2, where the parameterization is an element of the ansatz space. In contrast, the relative discrete L^2 error is 26% for $M_{max} = 5$.

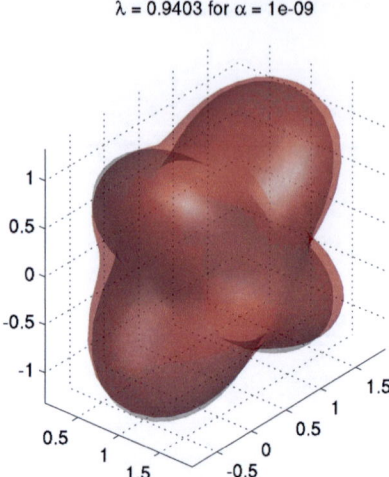

FIGURE 7.10. L^2 setting, $M_{\max} = 8$: Reconstruction (red) and original source (gray) after 50 gradient iterations. The relative discrete L^2 error is 18%.

CHAPTER 8

Conclusion and Outlook

In this thesis we introduce a geometric regularization method for bioluminescence tomography, which incorporates the *a priori* knowledge of piecewise constant sources and a Tikhonov like functional with a perimeter penalty term. Fundamental questions on the proposed scheme are answered in a general framework: existence of a solution, stability and regularization property are shown. Moreover, an analogous, self-contained theory for star-shaped sources is developed, as the star-shaped setting provides the necessary linear structure to apply optimization schemes.

In the second part the BLT problem based on the diffusion approximation is analyzed. Owing to the elliptic structure of the underlying partial differential equation, the domain derivative of the forward operator is well-known.[1] Based on the domain differentiability of the forward operator and the density of smooth shapes in the set of shapes with finite perimeter, an approximate variational principle is shown, which ensures the existence of smooth almost stationary shapes near the minimizing shape. This justifies the application of descent methods that converge to a stationary point in the reconstruction procedure. The discussion of the DA-based BLT problem is completed by testing numerically the geometric regularization scheme. Although incorporating *a priori* knowledge on the source via the admissible interval Λ and the regularization parameter α leads to

---

[1]Nevertheless, we present an elegant derivation of the domain derivative about a domain in Section 4.1.1.

useful reconstructions in some cases, the non-uniqueness of the DA-based BLT problem is a big challenge in all numerical experiments. In view of the uniqueness result for multispectral bioluminescence tomography in [**JW08**],[2] we think that the proposed geometric regularization method applied to multispectral BLT can counteract the observed issues. The theory in this work is easily transferred to the multispectral framework. It remains to verify the feasibility numerically. The generalization of the uniqueness result in multispectral BLT to star-shaped sources is another interesting open question.

The BLT problem based on the radiative transfer equation is investigated in the third part of this work. In contrast to the diffusion model, standard approaches cannot be applied for a rigorous derivation of the domain derivative of the forward operator. Nevertheless, we rigorously calculate the domain derivative about balls in the L^1 setting. The question is still open whether this result can be generalized to a larger class of domains rigorously. From a numerical point of view the proposed geometric regularization scheme works, even though the L^2 setting and the formal domain derivative about general star-shaped domains is used.[3] Due to the uniqueness of the RTE-based BLT problem with angularly resolved measurements, the sources are well reconstructed in all numerical experiments. However, there are two problems that may occur in practice but are not noticeable in our examples: First, when scattering is high and the object to be imaged is large, the measurements become diffuse, i.e., there is rarely any directional information in the boundary measurements, and we get in the regime of the diffusion model. Second, instead of angularly resolved measurements, angularly averaged data are often only available, which causes non-uniqueness of the BLT problem even based on the transport model. These two issues identify the need of additional independent source-measurement pairs and/or of cameras that also capture the directions of the photons in bioluminescence tomography. Former may be obtain by RTE-based multispectral BLT, which implies similar open questions as posed in the diffusion model above.

---

[2]Sources described by radial basis functions are uniquely determined by the boundary measurements, provided the optical parameters satisfy some assumptions. See [**JW08**] for details.

[3]We recall Remark 6.7 where we observe that the formal domain derivative is not an L^2 function. Consequently, the rigorous domain derivative does not exists in the L^2 setting.

Inspired by the recent trend of hybrid imaging methods, see [**AS12**] and the references therein, we suggest to couple bioluminescence tomography with a supplemental technique, in order to gain additional independent source-measurement pairs and to overcome the non-uniqueness problems. In particular, we think of utilizing the acousto-optic effect, which describes the influence of an acoustic wave on the optical properties and which is the basis for acousto-optic imaging, also known as ultrasound modulated optical tomography, cf. [**BS10, Bal13**], in bioluminescence tomography. Further work is required to develop and analyze the mathematical model of the 'coupled physics' technique and to verify its feasibility in practice.

We conclude that in special cases good reconstructions are obtained by the geometric regularization scheme. However, more research is needed to establish bioluminescence tomography as a reliable imaging technique for small animal models.

Appendices

APPENDIX A

Special Functions

In this chapter we present some results on special functions needed in this thesis. Although there exists a wide variety of literature on this topic, a few results are not given in the framework we consider here. Thus, we state them here explicitly and also the ideas to obtain them. Other results are presented for the sake of completeness only.

A.1. Legendre Functions

The following results on Legendre functions can be found in Chapter 5 of [**WG89**].

A.1.1. Legendre Polynomials. The polynomial solutions of the differential equation

$$(1 - x^2)y''(x) - 2xy'(x) + l(l+1)y(x) = 0 \quad \text{with } l \in \mathbb{N}_0$$

are called *Legendre polynomials.* The Legendre polynomial of degree $l \in \mathbb{N}_0$ is given by

$$P_l(x) = \frac{1}{2^l l!} \frac{\mathrm{d}}{\mathrm{d}x^l}(x^2 - 1)^l.$$

They satisfy the recurrence relation

$$(l+1)P_{l+1}(x) - (2l+1)xP_l(x) + lP_{l-1}(x) = 0 \tag{A.1}$$

for $l \in \mathbb{N}_0$. Here and in the following we use the convention that $P_{-1}(x) = 0$. The first three Legendre polynomial are

$$P_0(x) = 0 \,, \quad P_1(x) = x \,, \quad P_2(x) = \frac{1}{2}(3x^2 - 1) \,.$$

A.1.2. Associated Legendre Functions. For $m, l \in \mathbb{N}_0$ the functions $P_l^m \colon [-1, 1] \to \mathbb{R}$ with

$$P_l^m(x) = (-1)^m (1 - x^2)^{\frac{m}{2}} \frac{\mathrm{d}}{\mathrm{d}x} P_l(x)$$

are called *associated Legendre functions (of the first kind)* of degree l and order m.[1] We observe that P_l^m vanishes if $m > l$ and that $P_l^0 = P_l$. Moreover, the associated Legendre functions can be generalized to negative order and it holds

$$P_l^{-m} = (-1)^m \frac{(l-m)!}{(l+m)!} P_l^m \quad \text{for } m \in \mathbb{N} \,.$$

By differentiating the identity (A.1) the following recurrence relations are obtained, cf. [**WG89**, Section 5.13]:

$$(2l+1)x P_l^m(x) = (l+m) P_{l-1}^m(x) + (l-m+1) P_{l+1}^m(x) \,,$$
$$(2l+1)(1-x^2)^{\frac{1}{2}} P_l^m(x) = P_{l-1}^{m+1}(x) - P_{l+1}^{m+1}(x) \,. \tag{A.2}$$

Again, we finish this subsection by specifying the first three associated Legendre functions of non-vanishing order:

$$P_1^1(x) = -(1-x^2)^{\frac{1}{2}} \,, \quad P_2^1(x) = -3x(1-x^2)^{\frac{1}{2}} \,, \quad P_2^2(x) = 3(1-x^2) \,.$$

A.2. Spherical Harmonics

The restriction of harmonic homogeneous polynomials over $\mathbb{R}^d$ to the unit sphere $\Omega = S^{d-1}$ are called *spherical harmonics*. For the real-valued case in arbitrary space dimension $d \geq 2$ an overview of these functions can be found in [**AH12**]. Properties of complex-valued spherical harmonics in dimension 3 are presented in [**WG89**]. As we are mainly interested in the real-valued case in this thesis, we present some results in this setting in the following and transfer some results needed from the complex-valued framework to the real-valued. The books mentioned before are the main sources of this section, additional references are [**Hob55, Nat01b**].

---

[1]This is the definition of Hobson [**Hob55**, Chapter III]. In the literature there are sometimes different ones, e.g. with the term $(-1)^m$ missing.

A.2.1. In two Dimensions. Let

$$\omega = \begin{pmatrix} \cos\phi \\ \sin\phi \end{pmatrix} \in S^1 \quad \text{with } \phi \in [0, 2\pi[\,.$$

We will identify ω with ϕ and vice versa below. Then, the spherical harmonics of degree $l \in \mathbb{N}$ are linear combinations of

$$y_l^c(\omega) = \frac{1}{\sqrt{\pi}} \cos(l\phi) \quad \text{and} \quad y_l^s(\omega) = \frac{1}{\sqrt{\pi}} \sin(l\phi)$$

and the spherical harmonics of degree 0 are scalar multiples of

$$y_0 = \frac{1}{\sqrt{2\pi}}\,.$$

Moreover, the spherical harmonics are dense in $L^2(S^1)$ and the set

$$\{y_0\} \cup \{y_l^c : l \in \mathbb{N}\} \cup \{y_l^s : l \in \mathbb{N}\}$$

builds an orthonormal basis of $L^2(S^1)$, that is, for a function $f \in L^2(S^1)$ we have

$$f = \langle f, y_0 \rangle_{L^2} + \sum_{l=1}^{\infty} \left(\langle f, y_l^c \rangle_{L^2} y_l^c + \langle f, y_l^s \rangle_{L^2} y_l^s \right).$$

An useful result on spherical harmonics is the Funk–Hecke formula. Let $h \in C[-1, 1]$ and f_l a spherical harmonic of degree $l \in \mathbb{N}_0$. Then, the Funk–Hecke formula in dimension $d = 2$ reads

$$\int_{S^1} h(\omega \cdot \omega') f_l(\omega') \, d\omega' = \overline{h_l} f_l(\omega)\,. \tag{A.3}$$

Herein, the constant $\overline{h_l}$ is given by

$$\overline{h_l} = 2 \int_{-1}^{1} T_l(t) h(t) (1 - t^2)^{-\frac{1}{2}} \, dt$$

with T_l denoting the Chebyshev polynomial of degree l, i.e.,

$$T_l(t) = \cos(l \arccos t)\,.$$

A.2.2. In three Dimensions.
For $d = 3$ we identify a point $\omega \in \Omega = S^2$ with the pair of angles $(\vartheta, \phi) \in [0, \pi] \times [0, 2\pi[$ via

$$\omega = \begin{pmatrix} \cos\phi \sin\vartheta \\ \sin\phi \sin\vartheta \\ \cos\vartheta \end{pmatrix}\,.$$

There are $2l+1$ linearly independent spherical harmonics of degree $l \in \mathbb{N}_0$. A possible basis is build by

$$Y_{l,m}(\omega) = c_{l,m}P_l^m(\cos\vartheta)\cos(m\phi) \quad \text{for } m \in \{0, 1, \ldots, l\},$$
$$Y_{l,-m}(\omega) = c_{l,m}P_l^m(\cos\vartheta)\sin(m\phi) \quad \text{for } m \in \{1, 2, \ldots, l\}$$

with the choice

$$c_{l,0} = \sqrt{\frac{2l+1}{4\pi}} \quad \text{and} \quad c_{l,m} = \sqrt{\frac{2l+1}{2\pi}\frac{(l-m)!}{(l+m)!}}$$

in order to obtain an orthonormal basis with respect to the L^2 inner product. As in two dimensions, the spherical harmonics are dense in $L^2(S^2)$ and an orthonormal basis of $L^2(S^2)$ is given by

$$\{Y_{l,m} : l \in \mathbb{N}_0, m \in \mathbb{Z}, |m| \le l\}.$$

Hence, for every function $f \in L^2(S^2)$ holds

$$f = \sum_{l=0}^{\infty}\sum_{m=-l}^{l}\langle f, Y_{l,m}\rangle_{L^2}Y_{l,m}.$$

The Funk–Hecke formula also holds true for $d = 3$, because it is a space independent property of spherical harmonics. Only the constant $\overline{h_l}$ depends on the dimension d. Let $h \in C[-1, 1]$ and f_l be a spherical harmonic of degree $l \in \mathbb{N}_0$. Then,

$$\int_{S^2} h(\omega \cdot \omega') f_l(\omega')\, d\omega' = \overline{h_l} f_l(\omega) \qquad (A.4)$$

with

$$\overline{h_l} = 4\pi \int_{-1}^{1} h(t) P_l(t)\, dt.$$

In the derivation of the diffusion model from the transport model, to be more specific in Appendix B.1, we need recurrence relations for the real-valued spherical harmonics $Y_{l,m}$. To obtain them, we make a detour via the complex-valued spherical harmonics

$$H_{l,m}(\omega) = \sqrt{\frac{2l+1}{4\pi}\frac{(l-m)!}{(l+m)!}}P_l^m(\cos\vartheta)e^{im\phi} \quad \text{for } l \in \mathbb{N}_0, m \in \mathbb{Z}, |m| \le l.$$

If $|m| > l$ or $l = -1$ we set $Y_{l,m} = H_{l,m} = 0$, which is reasonable in view of $P_l^m = 0$ for $|m| > l$ and of the convention $P_{-1} = 0$. All results mentioned above also hold for the complex-valued spherical harmonics if the inner product is adapted correspondingly. The following recurrence relations for $H_{l,m}$ can be deduced from (A.2), cf. [**WG89**, Section 5.15]:

$$\cos \vartheta H_{l,m} = \alpha_{l,m} H_{l-1,m} + \alpha_{l+1,m} H_{l+1,m} \, ,$$

$$\sin \vartheta e^{i\phi} H_{l,m} = \beta_{l,-m} H_{l-1,m+1} - \beta_{l+1,m+1} H_{l+1,m+1} \, ,$$

$$\sin \vartheta e^{-i\phi} H_{l,m} = -\beta_{l,m} H_{l-1,m-1} + \beta_{l+1,-m+1} H_{l+1,m-1}$$

with

$$\alpha_{l,m} = \sqrt{\frac{(l+m)(l-m)}{(2l+1)(2l-1)}} \quad \text{and} \quad \beta_{l,m} = \sqrt{\frac{(l+m)(l+m-1)}{(2l+1)(2l-1)}} \, .$$

Using these relations as well as the identities $Y_{l,0} = H_{l,0}$ for $l \geq 0$ and

$$Y_{l,m} = \frac{1}{\sqrt{2}} \left(H_{l,m} + (-1)^m H_{l,-m} \right), \quad Y_{l,-m} = \frac{1}{i\sqrt{2}} \left(H_{l,m} - (-1)^m H_{l,-m} \right)$$

for $1 \leq m \leq l$, we can show by easy but technical calculations the recurrence formulae:

$$\cos \vartheta Y_{l,0} = \alpha_{l,0} Y_{l-1,0} + \alpha_{l+1,0} Y_{l+1,0} \, ,$$

$$\sin \vartheta \cos \phi Y_{l,0} = \frac{1}{\sqrt{2}} \left(\beta_{l,0} Y_{l-1,1} - \beta_{l+1,1} Y_{l+1,1} \right), \tag{A.5}$$

$$\sin \vartheta \sin \phi Y_{l,0} = \frac{1}{\sqrt{2}} \left(\beta_{l,0} Y_{l-1,-1} - \beta_{l+1,1} Y_{l+1,-1} \right)$$

for $l \in \mathbb{N}_0$, and for $l, m \in \mathbb{N}$

$$\cos \vartheta Y_{l,m} = \alpha_{l,m} Y_{l-1,m} + \alpha_{l+1,m} Y_{l+1,m} \, ,$$

$$\sin \vartheta \cos \phi Y_{l,m} = \frac{1}{2} \Big(\beta_{l,-m} Y_{l-1,m+1} - \beta_{l+1,m+1} Y_{l+1,m+1}$$

$$- \beta_{l,m} Y_{l-1,m-1} + \beta_{l+1,m+1} Y_{l+1,m-1} \Big), \tag{A.6}$$

$$\sin \vartheta \sin \phi Y_{l,m} = \frac{1}{2} \Big(\beta_{l,-m} Y_{l-1,-m-1} - \beta_{l+1,m+1} Y_{l+1,-m-1}$$

$$- \beta_{l,m} Y_{l-1,-m+1} + \beta_{l+1,-m+1} Y_{l+1,-m+1} \Big),$$

as well as

$$\cos \vartheta Y_{l,-m} = \alpha_{l,m} Y_{l-1,-m} + \alpha_{l+1,m} Y_{l+1,-m}\,,$$

$$\sin \vartheta \cos \phi Y_{l,-m} = \frac{1}{2}\Big(\beta_{l,-m} Y_{l-1,-m-1} - \beta_{l+1,m+1} Y_{l+1,-m-1}$$

$$- \beta_{l,m} Y_{l-1,-m+1} + \beta_{l+1,-m+1} Y_{l+1,-m+1}\Big)\,, \quad (A.7)$$

$$\sin \vartheta \sin \phi Y_{l,-m} = \frac{1}{2}\Big(\beta_{l,-m} Y_{l-1,m+1} - \beta_{l+1,m+1} Y_{l+1,m+1}$$

$$- \beta_{l,m} Y_{l-1,m-1} + \beta_{l+1,-m+1} Y_{l+1,m-1}\Big)\,.$$

Furthermore, the following addition theorem holds for both the real-valued and complex-valued spherical harmonics:

$$\sum_{m=-l}^{l} Y_{l,m}(\omega) Y_{l,m}(\theta) = \frac{2l+1}{4\pi} P_l(\omega \cdot \theta)\,,$$

$$\sum_{m=-l}^{l} H_{l,m}(\omega)\overline{H_{l,m}(\theta)} = \frac{2l+1}{4\pi} P_l(\omega \cdot \theta) \quad (A.8)$$

for $l \in \mathbb{N}_0$ and $\omega, \theta \in S^2$. Herein, P_l is the Legendre polynomial of degree l.

Let us finish this subsection by specifying the spherical harmonics of degree less than one:

$$Y_{0,0}(\omega) = \sqrt{\frac{1}{4\pi}}\,, \qquad\qquad Y_{1,0}(\omega) = \sqrt{\frac{3}{4\pi}}\cos \vartheta\,,$$

$$Y_{1,1}(\omega) = -\sqrt{\frac{3}{4\pi}}\sin \vartheta \cos \phi\,, \quad Y_{1,-1}(\omega) = -\sqrt{\frac{3}{4\pi}}\sin \vartheta \sin \phi\,. \quad (A.9)$$

A.3. Bessel Functions

In this section we define different kind of Bessel functions and recall a few properties of them. The main reference of this presentation is [**WG89**], however some results are taken from [**AS72**].

Bessel functions solve the Bessel equation

$$y''(x) + \frac{1}{x}y'(x) + \Big(1 - \frac{\nu^2}{x^2}\Big)y(x) = 0\,,$$

where $\nu \in \mathbb{R}$ is called order of the equation and of the function.[2] The *Bessel functions of the first kind of order* ν are given by

$$J_{\pm\nu}(x) = \sum_{k=0}^{\infty} \frac{(-1)^k}{k!} \frac{1}{\Gamma(\pm\nu + k + 1)} \left(\frac{x}{2}\right)^{2k\pm\nu} \qquad (A.10)$$

with the common Gamma function Γ, cf. [**WG89**]. We observe directly that J_ν is a smooth solution of the Bessel equation if $\nu \geq 0$. In contrast, the *Bessel function of the second kind of order* ν

$$N_\nu(x) = \frac{\cos(\nu\pi)J_\nu(x) - J_{-\nu}(x)}{\sin(\nu\pi)}$$

has a singularity at $x = 0$. It also solve the Bessel equation of order ν and is sometimes called *Neumann function*. Furthermore, the *Bessel functions of the third kind of order* ν are

$$H_\nu^{(1)} = J_\nu + iN_\nu \quad \text{and} \quad H_\nu^{(2)} = J_\nu - iN_\nu.$$

They are often called *Hankel functions of the first and second kind*, respectively, and have the same singular behavior at $x = 0$ as N_ν.

Inserting an imaginary variable, $x = it$ with $t \in \mathbb{R}$, into a Bessel function, we observe that this Bessel function then satisfies the differential equation

$$y''(t) + \frac{1}{t}y'(t) - \left(1 - \frac{\nu^2}{t^2}\right)y(t) = 0.$$

Such a differential equation is obtained when we write the diffusion equation in polar coordinates in two dimensions. This leads to the *modified Bessel functions of the first kind and second kind* defined by

$$I_\nu(x) = i^{-\nu}J_\nu(ix) \quad \text{and} \quad K_\nu(x) = \frac{\pi}{2}i^{\nu+1}H_\nu^{(1)}(ix)$$

for $x \in \mathbb{R}$, respectively. Former is smooth just like J_ν for $\nu \geq 0$ and latter has a singularity at $x = 0$.

For $n \in \mathbb{Z}$ the *spherical Bessel functions* are defined via

$$j_n(x) = \sqrt{\frac{\pi}{2x}}J_{n+1/2}(x) \quad \text{and} \quad h_n^{(1)}(x) = \sqrt{\frac{\pi}{2x}}H_{n+1/2}^{(1)}(x). \qquad (A.11)$$

The second mapping is also known as *spherical Hankel function of the first kind*. These functions satisfy the spherical Bessel equation

$$y''(x) + \frac{2}{x}y'(x) + \left(1 - \frac{n(n+1)}{x^2}\right)y(x) = 0.$$

---

[2]Also complex-valued orders ν can be considered, however we restrict ourselves to real-valued ones.

Again, we observe that for $n \in \mathbb{N}_0$ the function j_n is smooth and $h_n^{(1)}$ has a singularity at $x = 0$. The function $h_n^{(1)}$ admits the representation

$$h_n^{(1)}(x) = \frac{e^{ix}}{(ix)^{n+1}} \sum_{k=0}^{n} \frac{(n+k)!}{k!(n-k)!} \frac{1}{(-2ix)^k} . \tag{A.12}$$

The spherical Bessel functions have the following asymptotic behavior for $n \to \infty$:

$$j_n(x) = \frac{x^n}{1 \cdot 3 \cdots (2n+1)} \left(1 + O\left(\frac{1}{n}\right) \right) \tag{A.13}$$

uniformly on every compact subset of $\mathbb{C}$ and

$$h_n^{(1)}(x) = \frac{1 \cdot 3 \cdots (2n-1)}{ix^{n+1}} \left(1 + O\left(\frac{1}{n}\right) \right) \tag{A.14}$$

uniformly on every compact subset of $\mathbb{C}_+ = \{z \in \mathbb{C} \colon \operatorname{Re} z > 0, \operatorname{Im} z > 0\}$. The derivatives of j_n and $h_n^{(1)}$ satisfy the relations

$$
\begin{aligned}
j_n'(x) &= j_{n-1}(x) - \frac{n+1}{x} j_n(x) , \\
h_n^{(1)\prime}(x) &= h_{n-1}^{(1)}(x) - \frac{n+1}{x} h_n^{(1)}(x) .
\end{aligned} \tag{A.15}
$$

Moreover, the Wronskian of j_n and $h_n^{(1)}$ admits the form

$$j_n(x) h_n^{(1)\prime}(x) - j_n'(x) h_n^{(1)}(x) = \frac{i}{x^2} . \tag{A.16}$$

For $n = 0$ we have

$$j_0(x) = \frac{\sin x}{x} , \quad h_0^{(1)}(x) = \frac{-ie^{ix}}{x}$$

and, if $x = it, t \in \mathbb{R}$,

$$j_0(it) = \frac{\sinh t}{t} , \quad h_0^{(1)}(it) = \frac{-e^{-t}}{t} .$$

Supplements to the Derivation of the Diffusion Model

B.1. Some Calculations for the Case $d = 3$

In this section we calculate the integrals of ω needed in Subsection 2.1.2. From equation (A.9) we have a representation of $\omega \in \Omega = S^2$ by means of spherical harmonics of degree 1, namely

$$
\omega = \sqrt{\frac{4\pi}{3}} \begin{pmatrix} -Y_{1,1}(\omega) \\ -Y_{1,-1}(\omega) \\ Y_{1,0}(\omega) \end{pmatrix}.
$$

As the spherical harmonics $\{Y_{l,m} \colon l \in \mathbb{N}_0, m \in \mathbb{Z}, |m| \leq l\}$ build an orthonormal basis of $L^2(\Omega)$, we see immediately that

$$
\int_\Omega \omega \, d\omega = 0. \tag{B.1}
$$

By the same argument we obtain the identity

$$
\int_\Omega \omega\omega^T \, d\omega = \frac{4\pi}{3} \int_\Omega \begin{pmatrix} Y_{1,1}^2 & Y_{1,1}Y_{1,-1} & -Y_{1,1}Y_{1,0} \\ Y_{1,-1}Y_{1,1} & Y_{1,-1}^2 & Y_{1,-1}Y_{1,0} \\ -Y_{1,1}Y_{1,0} & -Y_{1,-1}Y_{1,0} & Y_{1,0}^2 \end{pmatrix} (\omega) \, d\omega \tag{B.2}
$$

$$
= \frac{4\pi}{3} I.
$$

Furthermore, we have, given any vector $a \in \mathbb{R}^3$, that

$$
\int_\Omega (\omega \cdot a)\omega\omega^T \, d\omega = 0. \tag{B.3}
$$

To show this, we rewrite the integrand as

$$(\omega \cdot a)\omega\omega^T = (\omega \cdot a) \begin{pmatrix} Y_{1,1} & 0 & 0 \\ 0 & Y_{1,-1} & 0 \\ 0 & 0 & Y_{1,0} \end{pmatrix} \begin{pmatrix} Y_{1,1} & Y_{1,-1} & -Y_{1,0} \\ Y_{1,1} & Y_{1,-1} & Y_{1,0} \\ -Y_{1,1} & -Y_{1,-1} & Y_{1,0} \end{pmatrix}$$

and the scalar factor as $\omega \cdot a = (a_1 \cos\phi \sin\vartheta + a_2 \sin\phi \sin\vartheta + a_3 \cos\vartheta)$. Using the recurrence formulae (A.5)-(A.7), we observe that the terms $(\omega \cdot a)Y_{1,m}$, $m \in \{-1, 0, 1\}$, are linear combinations of spherical harmonics of degree 0 and of degree 2. The statement follows immediately from the orthogonality of the spherical harmonics $Y_{l,m}$.

Moreover, the identities

$$\int_{\nu \cdot \omega < 0} \nu \cdot \omega \, d\omega = -\pi \quad \text{and} \quad \int_{\nu \cdot \omega < 0} (\nu \cdot \omega)\omega \, d\omega = \frac{2\pi}{3}\nu \qquad \text{(B.4)}$$

hold for $\nu \in \Omega$. To verify the first equation, we consider w.l.o.g. $\nu = e_3 = (0,0,1)^T$ and observe

$$\int_{e_3 \cdot \omega < 0} e_3 \cdot \omega \, d\omega = \int_0^{2\pi} \int_{\frac{\pi}{2}}^{\pi} \cos\vartheta \sin\vartheta \, d\vartheta \, d\phi = -\pi \, .$$

The second identity follows from some easy technical calculations that we only sketch here. If $\nu = e_1$, we see that

$$\int_{e_1 \cdot \omega < 0} (e_1 \cdot \omega)\omega \, d\omega = \int_{\pi}^{2\pi} \int_0^{\frac{\pi}{2}} \begin{pmatrix} \cos^2\phi \sin^3\vartheta \\ \cos\phi \sin\phi \sin^3\vartheta \\ \cos\phi \sin^2\vartheta \cos\vartheta \end{pmatrix} d\vartheta \, d\phi$$

$$+ \int_0^{\pi} \int_{\frac{\pi}{2}}^{\pi} \begin{pmatrix} \cos^2\phi \sin^3\vartheta \\ \cos\phi \sin\phi \sin^3\vartheta \\ \cos\phi \sin^2\vartheta \cos\vartheta \end{pmatrix} d\vartheta \, d\phi$$

$$= \frac{2\pi}{3}e_1 \, .$$

Similarly, we obtain the second identity of (B.4) for $\nu = e_2$ and $\nu = e_3$. Using the decomposition $\nu = \nu_1 e_1 + \nu_2 e_2 + \nu_3 e_3$, the second equation of (B.4) follows for general $\nu \in \Omega$.

B.2. Derivation of the Diffusion Model for $d = 2$

The derivation of the diffusion model for $d = 2$ is similar to the one for $d = 3$, however some constants differ. This is caused by the fact that the first moments of ω take different values. So in this section we mainly calculate the first moments of ω in case $d = 2$ and point out how these results affect the derivation of the diffusion model, as performed in Subsection 2.1.2 in case of $d = 3$.

Let $\omega \in \Omega = S^1$. Then we can express it in terms of spherical harmonics, namely

$$\omega = \begin{pmatrix} \cos \phi \\ \sin \phi \end{pmatrix} = \sqrt{\pi} \begin{pmatrix} y_1^c(\omega) \\ y_1^s(\omega) \end{pmatrix}.$$

By the orthogonality of the spherical harmonics we immediately observe

$$\int_\Omega \omega \, d\omega = 0 \tag{B.5}$$

and

$$\int_\Omega \omega \omega^T \, d\omega = \pi \int_\Omega \begin{pmatrix} (y_1^c)^2 & y_1^c y_1^s \\ y_1^c y_1^s & (y_1^s)^2 \end{pmatrix} (\omega) \, d\omega = \pi I. \tag{B.6}$$

Thus, the linear ansatz for $u(x, \cdot)$, cf. equation (2.9), reads for $d = 2$:

$$u(x, \omega) = u_0(x) + 2u_1(x) \cdot \omega. \tag{B.7}$$

By direct calculation we obtain

$$\begin{aligned} \int_\Omega (\omega \cdot a) \omega \omega^T \, d\omega &= \int_0^{2\pi} \begin{pmatrix} \cos^2 \phi & \cos \phi \sin \phi \\ \cos \phi \sin \phi & \sin^2 \phi \end{pmatrix} (a_1 \cos \phi + a_2 \sin \phi) \, d\phi \\ &= 0, \end{aligned}$$

which corresponds to (B.3) for $d = 3$. Using this and (B.6), we deduce as in Subsection 2.1.2 but with different constants the relation

$$(\nabla \cdot u_2)^T = \frac{1}{2} \nabla u_0.$$

All remaining steps in the derivation of the diffusion equation can be performed similar to the case $d = 3$ if we redefine the diffusion coefficient

$$D = \frac{1}{2(\sigma_a + \sigma_s')}. \tag{B.8}$$

This finally results in the identical looking diffusion approximation

$$-\nabla \cdot (D \nabla u_0) + \sigma_a u_0 = q \quad \text{in } X.$$

The next step is to adapt the boundary conditions. We will see that the difference in dimension becomes more apparent. The crucial part is the calculation of the integrals

$$\int_{\nu \cdot \omega < 0} \nu \cdot \omega \, d\omega = -2 \quad \text{and} \quad \int_{\nu \cdot \omega < 0} (\nu \cdot \omega) \omega \, d\omega = \frac{\pi}{2} \nu$$

with $\nu = (\cos\phi_\nu, \sin\phi_\nu)^T \in \Omega$. The first equation holds since

$$\int_{\nu \cdot \omega < 0} \nu \cdot \omega \, d\omega = \int_0^{2\pi} \cos\theta \chi_{\{\cos\theta < 0\}}(\theta) \, d\theta$$

$$= \int_{\frac{\pi}{2}}^{\frac{3\pi}{2}} \cos\theta \, d\theta = -2$$

via the substitution $\theta = \phi - \phi_\nu$. Applying the trigonometric identities

$$\cos(\phi - \phi_\nu)\cos\phi = \frac{1}{2}\left(\cos\phi_\nu + \cos(2\phi - \phi_\nu)\right)$$

and

$$\sin(\phi - \phi_\nu)\sin\phi = \frac{1}{2}\left(\sin\phi_\nu + \sin(2\phi - \phi_\nu)\right),$$

we find

$$\int_{\nu \cdot \omega < 0} (\nu \cdot \omega)\omega \, d\omega = \int_0^{2\pi} \cos(\phi - \phi_\nu)\chi_{\{\cos(\phi - \phi_\nu) < 0\}}(\phi) \begin{pmatrix} \cos\phi \\ \sin\phi \end{pmatrix} d\phi$$

$$= \frac{1}{2}\int_{\frac{\pi}{2}+\phi_\nu}^{\frac{3\pi}{2}+\phi_\nu} \begin{pmatrix} \cos\phi_\nu + \cos(2\phi - \phi_\nu) \\ \sin\phi_\nu + \sin(2\phi - \phi_\nu) \end{pmatrix} d\phi$$

$$= \frac{\pi}{2}\nu.$$

So the Robin boundary condition modeling the incoming flux, see (2.16) for the case $d = 3$, becomes

$$u_0 + \frac{\pi}{2}D\frac{\partial u_0}{\partial \nu} = 0 \quad \text{on } \partial X. \tag{B.9}$$

In contrast, the measurements look identical in both dimensions and correspond to the Neumann boundary values

$$D\frac{\partial u_0}{\partial \nu} = -g_0 \quad \text{on } \partial X. \tag{B.10}$$

However, we have to take note of the redefinition of the diffusion coefficient in (B.8).

APPENDIX C

Supplement to Section 6.2: Argument in Two Dimensions

In Section 6.2 the domain derivative of the RTE-based BLT forward operator is derived rigorously. However, the proofs of Theorem 6.6 and Lemma 6.11 are only performed in case $d = 3$. In this section we point out how to adapt these proofs in the case $d = 2$.

C.0.1. Adaption of the Proof of Theorem 6.6. In the proof of Theorem 6.6 the identities (6.18) and (6.19) are essentially the dimension depending observations. As in three dimensions, we consider the cases $x \in \Gamma$ and $x \in X \setminus \overline{\Gamma}$ separately.

Let $x \in \Gamma \setminus \{0\}$. In two dimensions, we have, instead of (6.18), the following identity:

$$\int_\Omega \frac{1}{|\omega \cdot \nu(p_1(x,\omega))|} \, \mathrm{d}\omega = R \int_\Omega \frac{1}{\sqrt{R^2 - (x^T \omega_\perp)^2}} \, \mathrm{d}\omega$$

$$= \frac{R}{|x|} \int_\Omega \left(\frac{R^2}{|x|^2} - \left(\left(\frac{x}{|x|}\right)^T \omega_\perp \right)^2 \right)^{-\frac{1}{2}} \, \mathrm{d}\omega_\perp$$

$$= 2\frac{R}{|x|} \int_{-1}^1 \left[\left(\frac{R^2}{|x|^2} - s^2 \right) \left(1 - s^2 \right) \right]^{-\frac{1}{2}} \, \mathrm{d}s \,,$$

where we use the change of variables $s = x^T \omega_\perp / |x|$, see again Section VII.2 in [**Nat01b**] for more details. We estimate the latter integral by

157

$$2\frac{R}{|x|}\int_{-1}^{1}\left[\left(\frac{R^2}{|x|^2}-s^2\right)(1-s^2)\right]^{-\frac{1}{2}}ds$$

$$=4\frac{R}{|x|}\int_{0}^{1}\left[\left(\frac{R}{|x|}-s\right)\left(\frac{R}{|x|}+s\right)(1-s)(1+s)\right]^{-\frac{1}{2}}ds$$

$$\leq 4\sqrt{\frac{R}{|x|}}\int_{0}^{1}\left[s^2-\left(\frac{R}{|x|}+1\right)s+\frac{R}{|x|}\right]^{-\frac{1}{2}}ds.$$

The primitive of the integrand in the last line is known and it follows that

$$2\frac{R}{|x|}\int_{-1}^{1}\left[\left(\frac{R^2}{|x|^2}-s^2\right)(1-s^2)\right]^{-\frac{1}{2}}ds$$

$$\leq 4\sqrt{\frac{R}{|x|}}\ln\left(2\sqrt{s^2-\left(\frac{R}{|x|}+1\right)s+\frac{R}{|x|}}+2s-\frac{R}{|x|}-1\right)\Bigg|_{0}^{1}$$

$$=4\sqrt{\frac{R}{|x|}}\ln\left(\frac{R-|x|}{R+|x|-2\sqrt{R|x|}}\right)$$

$$=4\sqrt{\frac{R}{|x|}}\ln\left(\frac{\sqrt{R}+\sqrt{|x|}}{\sqrt{R}-\sqrt{|x|}}\right)$$

$$=4\sqrt{\frac{R}{|x|}}\ln\left(\frac{R+|x|+2\sqrt{R|x|}}{R-|x|}\right)$$

$$=4\sqrt{\frac{R}{|x|}}\left[\ln\left(R+|x|+2\sqrt{R|x|}\right)-\ln\left(R-|x|\right)\right].$$

The expression on the right-hand side is integrable in x over Γ, since the integrals

$$\int_{0}^{R}\rho^{-\frac{1}{2}}\,d\rho=2\sqrt{R}\quad\text{and}\quad\int_{0}^{R}\ln(R-\rho)\,d\rho=R(\ln R-1)$$

exist. Thus, we have an integrable upper bound of the absolute momentum $\overline{H}$. We conclude that

$$H|_{\Gamma\times\Omega}\in L^1(X\times\Omega)\quad\text{with}\quad\|H|_{\Gamma\times\Omega}\|_{L^1}\leq C_1\|h_\nu\|_\infty,$$

where the constant C_1 only depends on R.

Now let $x \in X \setminus \overline{\Gamma}$. In place of (6.19), we have in two dimensions the identity

$$\int_\Omega \frac{\psi(x,\omega)}{|\omega \cdot \nu(p_i(x,\omega))|}\, d\omega = R \int_{x^T\omega_\perp \in]-R,R[} \frac{1}{\sqrt{R^2 - (x^T\omega_\perp)^2}}\, d\omega_\perp$$

$$= R \int_{\arccos(\frac{R}{|x|})}^{\arccos(-\frac{R}{|x|})} \frac{1}{\sqrt{R^2 - (|x|\cos\phi)^2}}\, d\phi$$

$$= R \int_{-\frac{R}{|x|}}^{\frac{R}{|x|}} \left(\left(R^2 - |x|^2 s^2\right)\left(1 - s^2\right) \right)^{-\frac{1}{2}} ds,$$

where we first use the parameterization $\omega_\perp(\phi)$ of the sphere Ω such that $x^T\omega_\perp = |x|\cos\phi$ and second the change of variables $s = \cos\phi$. The integral can be estimated by

$$R \int_{-\frac{R}{|x|}}^{\frac{R}{|x|}} \left(\left(R^2 - |x|^2 s^2\right)\left(1 - s^2\right) \right)^{-\frac{1}{2}} ds$$

$$= 2R \int_0^{\frac{R}{|x|}} \left(\left(R + |x|s\right)\left(1 + s\right)\left(R - |x|s\right)\left(1 - s\right) \right)^{-\frac{1}{2}} ds$$

$$\leq 2\sqrt{R} \int_0^{\frac{R}{|x|}} \left(|x|s^2 - \left(R + |x|\right)s + R \right)^{-\frac{1}{2}} ds.$$

Proceeding similar to the calculations above, we obtain

$$2\sqrt{R} \int_0^{\frac{R}{|x|}} \left(|x|s^2 - \left(R + |x|\right)s + R \right)^{-\frac{1}{2}} ds$$

$$= 2\sqrt{\frac{R}{|x|}} \ln\left(\sqrt{|x|^2 s^2 - \left(R + |x|\right)|x|s + R|x|} + 2|x|s - R - |x| \right)\Big|_0^{\frac{R}{|x|}}$$

$$= 2\sqrt{\frac{R}{|x|}} \left[\ln\left(R + |x| + 2\sqrt{R|x|} \right) - \ln\left(|x| - R \right) \right],$$

which is integrable in x over $X \setminus \overline{\Gamma}$. In addition, the integral only depends on R and its value is denoted by C_2. It follows that

$$H|_{(X\setminus\overline{\Gamma})\times\Omega} \in L^1(X \times \Omega) \quad \text{with} \quad \|H|_{(X\setminus\overline{\Gamma})\times\Omega}\|_{L^1} \leq C_2\|h_\nu\|_\infty.$$

Combining the estimates obtained in both cases, we finally obtain that, also in case $d = 2$, $H \in L^1(X \times \Omega)$ with

$$\|H\|_{L^1} \leq C\|h_\nu\|_\infty.$$

Herein, $C = \max\{C_1, C_2\}$.

Remark C.1. We note that, in contrast to the findings in three dimensions, the function $\overline{H}$ is not essentially bounded in X in two dimensions. We only have that $\overline{H}$ is integrable over X. Nevertheless, this result is sufficient to obtain the statement of Theorem 6.6 and also of Lemma 6.11 in the upcoming paragraph.

C.0.2. Adaption of the Proof of Lemma 6.11.

In order to prove Lemma 6.11 in two dimensions, we have to reconsider the estimates (6.20) and (6.21) as well as (6.23)-(6.25).

In Remark C.1 we noticed that, in contrast to (6.20), we have no essential upper bound of

$$\int_\Omega \psi(x,\omega) \frac{1}{\left|\omega \cdot \nu\bigl(p_i(x,\omega)\bigr)\right|}\, d\omega$$

in case $d = 2$. However, we know from the previous section that there exists a constant $C > 0$ such that

$$\int_X \int_\Omega \psi(x,\omega) \frac{1}{\left|\omega \cdot \nu\bigl(p_i(x,\omega)\bigr)\right|}\, d\omega\, dx \leq C\,.$$

Using this estimate, we obtain similar to (6.21) and (6.23):

$$\left\|(f_h - f)\chi_{\Gamma \cap \Gamma_h}\right\|_{L^1} \leq 3C\|h_\nu\|_\infty\,,$$

$$\int_X \int_\Omega \psi(x,\omega)\psi_h(x,\omega)\bigl|f_h(x,\omega) - f(x,\omega)\bigr|\, d\omega\, dx \leq 6C\|h_\nu\|_\infty\,.$$

It remains to show that the expressions on the left-hand side of (6.24) and (6.25) are integrable over $X \setminus (\overline{\Gamma \cup \Gamma_h})$. Let $x \in X \setminus (\overline{\Gamma \cup \Gamma_h})$. We begin deriving a two-dimensional analog to (6.24). From (6.24) we know that

$$\int_\Omega \psi(x,\omega)\bigl(1 - \psi_h(x,\omega)\bigr)\bigl|f_h(x,\omega) - f(x,\omega)\bigr|\, d\omega$$

$$\leq \int_\Omega \psi(x,\omega)\bigl(1 - \psi_h(x,\omega)\bigr)\bigl|\tau_1(x,\omega) - \tau_2(x,\omega)\bigr|\, d\omega$$

$$\leq 4\sqrt{2\|h_\nu\|_\infty R - \|h_\nu\|_\infty^2} \int_{x^T\omega_\perp \in [R - \|h_\nu\|_\infty, R[} 1\, d\omega_\perp\,.$$

Using once more the parameterization $\omega_\perp(\phi)$ with $x^T\omega_\perp = |x|\cos\phi$, we observe

$$\int_{x^T\omega_\perp\in[R-\|h_\nu\|_\infty,R[} 1\,\mathrm{d}\omega_\perp = \int_{\arccos(\frac{R}{|x|})}^{\arccos(\frac{R-\|h_\nu\|_\infty}{|x|})} \mathrm{d}\phi$$

$$= \arccos\Big(\frac{R-\|h_\nu\|_\infty}{|x|}\Big) - \arccos\Big(\frac{R}{|x|}\Big).$$

Application of the mean value theorem yields

$$\arccos\Big(\frac{R-\|h_\nu\|_\infty}{|x|}\Big) - \arccos\Big(\frac{R}{|x|}\Big) \le \Big(1 - \Big(\frac{R}{|x|}\Big)^2\Big)^{-\frac{1}{2}} \frac{\|h_\nu\|_\infty}{|x|}$$

$$= \frac{\|h_\nu\|_\infty}{\sqrt{|x|^2 - R^2}}.$$

The term on the right-hand side is integrable in x over $X\setminus\overline{\Gamma}$ in view of

$$\int_R^M \frac{1}{\sqrt{\rho^2 - R^2}}\,\mathrm{d}\rho = \ln\Big(M + \sqrt{M^2 - R^2}\Big) - \ln R \quad \text{for } M > R. \quad \text{(C.1)}$$

Consequently, there exists a constant C_1 depending only on R such that

$$\int_{X\setminus(\overline{\Gamma\cup\Gamma_h})} \int_\Omega \psi(x,\omega)\big(1 - \psi_h(x,\omega)\big)\big|f_h(x,\omega) - f(x,\omega)\big|\,\mathrm{d}\omega\,\mathrm{d}x$$

$$\le C_1\|h_\nu\|_\infty^{\frac{3}{2}}\sqrt{2R - \|h_\nu\|_\infty}\,.$$

In exactly the same manner we also find a constant $C_2 > 0$, but now depending on R and $\|h_\nu\|_\infty$, with

$$\int_{X\setminus(\overline{\Gamma\cup\Gamma_h})} \int_\Omega \big(1 - \psi(x,\omega)\big)\psi_h(x,\omega)\big|f_h(x,\omega) - f(x,\omega)\big|\,\mathrm{d}\omega\,\mathrm{d}x$$

$$\le C_2\|h_\nu\|_\infty^{\frac{3}{2}}\sqrt{2R + \|h_\nu\|_\infty}\,,$$

which is (6.25) revisited. We point out that the constant C_2 converges to C_1 as $h \to 0$, since the integral (C.1) is continuous with respect to R.

Finally, we have all necessary adaptions to the two-dimensional situation at hand. By a combination of the adapted findings, obtained in this appendix, with the dimension independent results in the proof of Lemma 6.11, we verify the statement in case $d = 2$.

APPENDIX D

Singular Value Decomposition of the Linear DA-based BLT Forward Operator

---

In this chapter we derive the singular value decomposition of the linear DA-based BLT forward operator A, defined in (2.30), in the special case of a ball-shaped domain $X \subset \mathbb{R}^3$ and constant coefficients D, σ_{a}. In addition, we investigate the asymptotic behavior of the singular values. These results allow to gain an insight into the ill-posedness of the BLT problem in the DA-framework: Not only the decay of the singular values describe the order of ill-posedness, but also the singular functions indicate which sources can be reconstructed at all.

Before we state the two main results of this chapter, namely the singular value decomposition of A and the asymptotic behavior of the singular values, we begin with a short summary of notations and results that we need in the proof. They are either known from the previous chapters or easy observations.

Let us recall some definitions from Section 2.2.2. The linear forward operator of DA-based BLT is given by

$$A\colon L^2(X) \to L^2(\partial X), \quad q \mapsto u|_{\partial X}, \qquad \text{(D.1)}$$

where $u \in H^1(X)$ is the weak solution of the boundary value problem

$$-\mathrm{div}\big(D\nabla u\big) + \sigma_{\mathrm{a}} u = q \quad \text{in } X,$$

$$u + 2D\frac{\partial u}{\partial \nu} = 0 \quad \text{on } \partial X. \qquad \text{(D.2)}$$

More precisely, u solves the variational equation

$$\int_X (D\nabla u \cdot \nabla v + \sigma_a uv)\,\mathrm{d}x + \frac{1}{2}\int_{\partial X} uv\,\mathrm{d}\mu = \int_X qv\,\mathrm{d}x \quad \forall v \in H^1(X). \quad (\text{D.3})$$

The adjoint of A is the operator

$$A^* : L^2(\partial X) \to L^2(X), \quad \psi \mapsto 2w, \quad (\text{D.4})$$

where $w \in H^1(X)$ is the weak solution of the adjoint boundary value problem

$$-\mathrm{div}\big(D\nabla w\big) + \sigma_a w = 0 \quad \text{in } X,$$
$$w + 2D\frac{\partial w}{\partial \nu} = \psi \quad \text{on } \partial X. \quad (\text{D.5})$$

This is easily observed from

$$\langle Aq, \psi\rangle_{L^2} = \int_{\partial X} u\psi\,\mathrm{d}\mu = 2\int_X (D\nabla u \cdot \nabla w + \sigma_a uw)\,\mathrm{d}x + \int_{\partial X} uw\,\mathrm{d}\mu$$
$$= 2\int_X qw\,\mathrm{d}x = \langle q, 2w\rangle_{L^2},$$

where the second identity is due to the weak formulation of the adjoint boundary value problem (D.5):

$$\int_X (D\nabla w \cdot \nabla v + \sigma_a wv)\,\mathrm{d}x + \frac{1}{2}\int_{\partial X} uv\,\mathrm{d}\mu = \frac{1}{2}\int_{\partial X} \psi v\,\mathrm{d}x \quad \forall v \in H^1(X).$$

As from now, we assume that $X \subset \mathbb{R}^3$ is the three-dimensional ball with radius $R > 0$ centered w.l.o.g. in the origin, i.e., $X = B_R(0)$. In addition, let D and σ_a be positive constants. For this special case, the fundamental solution of the diffusion equation is derived in Example 2.11. It is given by

$$\Phi(x,y) = \frac{e^{-\tilde{\sigma}|x-y|}}{4\pi D|x-y|} \quad \text{for } x \neq y \text{ with } \tilde{\sigma} = \sqrt{\frac{\sigma_a}{D}}$$

and has the representation

$$\Phi(x,y) = -\frac{\tilde{\sigma}}{D}\sum_{l=0}^{\infty}\sum_{m=-l}^{l} h_l^{(1)}(\tilde{\sigma}i|x|)H_{l,m}(\hat{x})j_l(\tilde{\sigma}i|y|)\overline{H_{l,m}(\hat{y})} \quad (\text{D.6})$$

for $|x| > |y|$ and with $\hat{x} = x/|x|$ as well as $\hat{y} = y/|y|$, see (2.31). Herein, $h_l^{(1)}$, j_l and $H_{l,m}$ are the spherical Hankel function of first kind, the spherical Bessel function and the complex-valued spherical harmonic, respectively, see Appendix A. We recall that the series in (D.6) converges absolutely and uniformly on compact subsets of $\{(x,y) \in \mathbb{R}^3 \times \mathbb{R}^3 : |x| > |y|\}$

and that this statement is also true for the series of the term by term derivatives with respect to $|x|$ and $|y|$.

Proceeding similar to Example 3.11, where the case $D = \sigma_{\mathrm{a}} = 1$ is considered, we obtain a Green's function of the boundary value problem (D.2) with arbitrary positive constants D and σ_{a}: Let

$$\phi(x,y) = \frac{\widetilde{\sigma}}{D} \sum_{l=0}^{\infty} \sum_{k=-l}^{l} \phi_{l,k}(y) j_l(\widetilde{\sigma}i|x|) H_{l,k}(\widehat{x}) \tag{D.7}$$

with

$$\phi_{l,k}(y) = \frac{2\widetilde{\sigma}i h_l^{(1)\prime}(\widetilde{\sigma}iR) + h_l^{(1)}(\widetilde{\sigma}iR)}{2\widetilde{\sigma}i j_l'(\widetilde{\sigma}iR) + j_l(\widetilde{\sigma}iR)} j_l(\widetilde{\sigma}i|y|) \overline{H_{l,k}(\widehat{y})} \,.$$

Then, the function

$$G(x,y) = \Phi(x,y) + \phi(x,y)$$

is a Green's function. We note that the series in (D.7) converges absolutely and uniformly on every compact subset of $\overline{X} \times X$.

The Green's function G can also be expanded in terms of real-valued spherical harmonics $Y_{l,m}$. From the addition formula (A.8) we have

$$\sum_{k=-l}^{l} H_{l,k}(\widehat{x}) \overline{H_{l,k}(\widehat{y})} = \sum_{k=-l}^{l} Y_{l,k}(\widehat{x}) Y_{l,k}(\widehat{y}) \,.$$

Consequently, G can be rewritten for $|x| > |y|$ as

$$G(x,y) = \sum_{l=0}^{\infty} \sum_{k=-l}^{l} g_l(|x|,|y|) Y_{l,k}(\widehat{x}) Y_{l,k}(\widehat{y}) \,, \tag{D.8}$$

where

$$g_l(|x|,|y|)$$
$$= \frac{\widetilde{\sigma}}{D} \left(\frac{2\widetilde{\sigma}i h_l^{(1)\prime}(\widetilde{\sigma}iR) + h_l^{(1)}(\widetilde{\sigma}iR)}{2\widetilde{\sigma}i j_l'(\widetilde{\sigma}iR) + j_l(\widetilde{\sigma}iR)} j_l(\widetilde{\sigma}i|x|) - h_l^{(1)}(\widetilde{\sigma}i|x|) \right) j_l(\widetilde{\sigma}i|y|) \,.$$

By means of the Green's function, the operator A and its adjoint A^* admit the following representations:

$$(Aq)(y) = \int_X q(x) G(y,x) \, \mathrm{d}x \qquad \text{for } y \in \partial X \,, \tag{D.9}$$

$$(A^*\psi)(x) = \int_{\partial X} \psi(y) G(y,x) \, \mathrm{d}\mu(y) \qquad \text{for } x \in X \,. \tag{D.10}$$

Former identity is a direct consequence of Green's representation formula, cf. (3.15). The latter relation holds, since

$$\langle Aq, \psi \rangle_{L^2} = \int_{\partial X} Aq(y)\psi(y)\,\mathrm{d}\mu(y) = \int_{\partial X}\int_X q(x)G(y,x)\,\mathrm{d}x\,\mathrm{d}\mu(y)$$

$$= \int_X q(x)\int_{\partial X} G(y,x)\psi(y)\,\mathrm{d}\mu(y)\,\mathrm{d}x = \langle q, A^*\psi\rangle_{L^2}\,.$$

After these preliminaries, we are now able to state the two main results of this chapter. The first characterizes the singular value decomposition of the DA-based BLT forward operator A under the above mentioned assumptions on D, σ_{a} and X.

Theorem D.1 (Singular Value Decomposition of A). *Let* $X = B_R(0)$, $R > 0$, *and* D, σ_{a} *be positive constants. Then, the operator* A *defined in* (D.1) *admits the singular system* $\big\{(\varsigma_l; \xi_{l,k}, \eta_{l,k})\colon l \in \mathbb{N}_0, k = -l,\dots,l\big\}$ *given by*

$$\varsigma_l = \beta_l R\frac{\widetilde{\sigma}}{D}\left(\frac{2\widetilde{\sigma}i h_l^{(1)\prime}(\widetilde{\sigma}iR) + h_l^{(1)}(\widetilde{\sigma}iR)}{2\widetilde{\sigma}i j_l'(\widetilde{\sigma}iR) + j_l(\widetilde{\sigma}iR)}j_l(\widetilde{\sigma}iR) - h_l^{(1)}(\widetilde{\sigma}iR)\right),$$

$$\xi_{l,k}(x) = \frac{1}{\beta_l}j_l(\widetilde{\sigma}i|x|)Y_{l,k}(\widehat{x})\,, \quad x \in X\,,$$

$$\eta_{l,k}(y) = \frac{1}{R}Y_{l,k}(\widehat{y})\,, \quad y \in \partial X\,,$$

where

$$\widetilde{\sigma} = \sqrt{\frac{\sigma_{\mathrm{a}}}{D}} \quad and \quad \beta_l = \left(\int_0^R j_l(\widetilde{\sigma}ir)^2 r^2\,\mathrm{d}r\right)^{\frac{1}{2}}.$$

PROOF. Before we start with the actual proof, we point out that the singular values ς_l are positive for $l \in \mathbb{N}_0$. This is observed recalling the definition of the spherical Bessel functions j_l, $h_l^{(1)}$ in (A.11) and the identities (A.10), (A.12), (A.15).

To show the statement, we have to verify the following four points: $A\xi_{l,k} = \varsigma_l\eta_{l,k}$, $A^*\eta_{l,k} = \varsigma_l\xi_{l,k}$, $\{\xi_{l,k}\colon l,k\}$ is a complete orthonormal system of $\mathcal{N}(A)^{\perp}$ and $\{\eta_{l,k}\colon l,k\}$ is a complete orthonormal system of $\overline{\mathcal{R}(A)}$.

We start showing that $A\xi_{l,k} = \varsigma_l\eta_{l,k}$. Let $l \in \mathbb{N}_0$, $k \in \{-l,\dots,l\}$ and $y \in \partial X = \partial B_R(0)$. Using the identity (D.9) and the expansion (D.8) of

G, we obtain

$$
A\xi_{l,k}(y) = \int_X \xi_{l,k}(x)G(y,x)\,\mathrm{d}x
$$

$$
= \int_X \xi_{l,k}(x)\sum_{m=0}^{\infty}\sum_{n=-m}^{m} g_m(R,|x|)Y_{m,n}(\widehat{y})Y_{m,n}(\widehat{x})\,\mathrm{d}x\,.
$$

A change of variables and the orthonormality of the spherical harmonics yield

$$
A\xi_{l,k}(y) = \int_0^R \int_{S^2}\sum_{m=0}^{\infty}\sum_{n=-m}^{m} \xi_{l,k}(r\theta)g_m(R,r)Y_{m,n}(\widehat{y})Y_{m,n}(\widehat{x})r^2\,\mathrm{d}\theta\,\mathrm{d}r
$$

$$
= \frac{1}{\beta_l}\int_0^R r^2 j_l(\widetilde{\sigma}ir)\left[\sum_{m=0}^{\infty}\sum_{n=-m}^{m} g_m(R,r)\int_{S^2} Y_{l,k}(\theta)Y_{m,n}(\theta)\,\mathrm{d}\theta\,Y_{m,n}(\widehat{y})\right]\mathrm{d}r
$$

$$
= \frac{1}{\beta_l}\left(\int_0^R r^2 j_l(\widetilde{\sigma}ir)g_l(R,r)r^2\,\mathrm{d}r\right)Y_{l,k}(\widehat{y})
$$

$$
= \frac{\widetilde{\sigma}}{D}\left(\frac{2\widetilde{\sigma}ih_l^{(1)\prime}(\widetilde{\sigma}iR)+h_l^{(1)}(\widetilde{\sigma}iR)}{2\widetilde{\sigma}ij_l'(\widetilde{\sigma}iR)+j_l(\widetilde{\sigma}iR)}j_l(\widetilde{\sigma}iR)-h_l^{(1)}(\widetilde{\sigma}iR)\right)\beta_l Y_{l,k}(\widehat{y})
$$

$$
= \varsigma_l \eta_{l,k}(y)\,.
$$

Next, we verify in a similar manner that $A^*\eta_{l,k} = \varsigma_l \xi_{l,k}$. Let $l \in \mathbb{N}_0$, $k \in \{-l,\ldots,l\}$ and $x \in X$. In view of the equations (D.10) and (D.8), we observe

$$
A^*\eta_{l,k}(x) = \int_{\partial X} \eta_{l,k}(y)G(y,x)\,\mathrm{d}\mu(y)
$$

$$
= \int_{\partial X} \eta_{l,k}(y)\sum_{m=0}^{\infty}\sum_{n=-m}^{m} g_m(R,|x|)Y_{m,n}(\widehat{y})Y_{m,n}(\widehat{x})\,\mathrm{d}\mu(y)\,.
$$

By the same arguments as above follows

$$
A^*\eta_{l,k}(x) = \frac{1}{R}\int_{\partial X}\sum_{m=0}^{\infty}\sum_{n=-m}^{m} Y_{l,k}(\widehat{y})g_m(R,|x|)Y_{m,n}(\widehat{y})Y_{m,n}(\widehat{x})\,\mathrm{d}\mu(y)
$$

$$
= \frac{1}{R}\sum_{m=0}^{\infty}\sum_{n=-m}^{m}\left[\int_{S^2} R^2 g_m(R,|x|)Y_{l,k}(\theta)Y_{m,n}(\theta)\,\mathrm{d}\theta\right]Y_{m,n}(\widehat{x})
$$

$$
= R\frac{\widetilde{\sigma}}{D}\left(\frac{2\widetilde{\sigma}ih_l^{(1)\prime}(\widetilde{\sigma}iR)+h_l^{(1)}(\widetilde{\sigma}iR)}{2\widetilde{\sigma}ij_l'(\widetilde{\sigma}iR)+j_l(\widetilde{\sigma}iR)}j_l(\widetilde{\sigma}iR)-h_l^{(1)}(\widetilde{\sigma}iR)\right)j_l(\widetilde{\sigma}i|x|)Y_{l,k}(\widehat{x})
$$

$$
= \varsigma_l \xi_{l,k}(x)\,.
$$

To finish the proof, it remains to show that $\{\eta_{l,k} : l \in \mathbb{N}_0, k = -l, \ldots, l\}$ is a complete orthonormal system of $\overline{\mathcal{R}(A)}$ and $\{\xi_{l,k} : l \in \mathbb{N}_0, k = -l, \ldots, l\}$ is a complete orthonormal system of $\mathcal{N}(A)^\perp$. It is well known, see also Appendix A.2, that the spherical harmonics $\{Y_{l,k} : l \in \mathbb{N}_0, k = -l, \ldots, l\}$ build an orthonormal basis of $L^2(S^2)$. With the transformation $\theta = y/R$, $y \in \partial X = \partial B_R(0)$, we obtain the completeness and orthonormality of $\{\eta_{l,k} : l \in \mathbb{N}_0, k = -l, \ldots, l\}$ in $L^2(\partial X)$. This space is exactly the closure of the range of A, since $\mathcal{R}(A) = H^{3/2}(\partial X)$, in the sense of set-theory, due to regularity theorems for elliptic boundary value problems, see [**Hac92**] for instance.

The completeness of $\{\xi_{l,k} : l \in \mathbb{N}_0, k = -l, \ldots, l\}$ in $\mathcal{N}(A)^\perp$ follows directly from the identity $\mathcal{N}(A)^\perp = \overline{\mathcal{R}(A^*)}$, see for instance [**Wer07**], the relation $\varsigma_l \xi_{l,k} = A^* \eta_{l,k}$ and the completeness of $\{\eta_{l,k} : l, k\}$ in $L^2(\partial X)$. Further, the set $\{\xi_{l,k} : l, k\}$ builds an orthonormal system, since

$$\langle \xi_{l,k}, \xi_{m,n} \rangle_{L^2(X)} = \frac{1}{\varsigma_l \varsigma_m} \langle A^* \eta_{l,k}, A^* \eta_{m,n} \rangle_{L^2(X)} = \frac{1}{\varsigma_l \varsigma_m} \langle A A^* \eta_{l,k}, \eta_{m,n} \rangle_{L^2(\partial X)}$$

$$= \frac{\varsigma_l}{\varsigma_m} \langle \eta_{l,k}, \eta_{m,n} \rangle_{L^2(\partial X)} = \delta_{l,m} \delta_{k,n} .$$

Herein, $\delta_{l,m}$ denotes the Kronecker delta. □

Let us point out that the non-uniqueness of the DA-based BLT problem, stated in Lemma 2.10, becomes apparent in the singular functions. Only linear combinations of the functions $j_l(\widetilde{\sigma} i |x|) Y_{l,k}(\widehat{x})$, which are fixed couplings of the radial and angular component, lie in the orthogonal complement of $\mathcal{N}(A)$ and can, therefore, be reconstructed. As soon as there is a different composition of the radial and angular component in the source, only the part having the above form can be reconstructed.

The second main result of this chapter gives an answer to the order of ill-posedness of the DA-based BLT problem. It characterizes the asymptotic decay of the singular values.

Theorem D.2 (Asymptotic behavior of ς_l). *Let the assumptions of Theorem D.1 hold. Then, the singular values ς_l of A have the asymptotic behavior*

$$\varsigma_l = \frac{2R^{\frac{3}{2}}}{D(2l+3)^{\frac{1}{2}}(2l+1)} \left[\frac{1 + O(l^{-1})}{1 + O(l^{-1})} \right] \quad as\ l \to \infty . \tag{D.11}$$

PROOF. From Theorem D.1 the singular values of A are known to be

$$\varsigma_l = \beta_l R \frac{\widetilde{\sigma}}{D} \left(\frac{2\widetilde{\sigma} i h_l^{(1)'}(\widetilde{\sigma} i R) + h_l^{(1)}(\widetilde{\sigma} i R)}{2\widetilde{\sigma} i j_l'(\widetilde{\sigma} i R) + j_l(\widetilde{\sigma} i R)} j_l(\widetilde{\sigma} i R) - h_l^{(1)}(\widetilde{\sigma} i R) \right) \tag{D.12}$$

with

$$\widetilde{\sigma} = \sqrt{\frac{\sigma_a}{D}} \quad \text{and} \quad \beta_l = \left(\int_0^R j_l(\widetilde{\sigma}ir)^2 r^2 \, dr \right)^{\frac{1}{2}}.$$

In a first step, we calculate the asymptotic behavior of the term in parentheses in (D.12). According to (A.16), the Wronskian of j_l and $h_l^{(1)}$ satisfies

$$j_l(z)h_l^{(1)\prime}(z) - j_l'(z)h_l^{(1)}(z) = \frac{i}{z^2}.$$

Hence,

$$\left(2\widetilde{\sigma}ih_l^{(1)\prime}(\widetilde{\sigma}iR) + h_l^{(1)}(\widetilde{\sigma}iR) \right) j_l(\widetilde{\sigma}iR) - \left(2\widetilde{\sigma}ij_l'(\widetilde{\sigma}iR) + j_l(\widetilde{\sigma}iR) \right) h_l^{(1)}(\widetilde{\sigma}iR)$$

$$= \frac{2}{\widetilde{\sigma}R^2}.$$

Dividing by $2\widetilde{\sigma}ij_l'(\widetilde{\sigma}iR) + j_l(\widetilde{\sigma}iR)$ and estimating this term will yield the asymptotic behavior of the term in parentheses. We recall from (A.15) that

$$j_l'(\widetilde{\sigma}iR) = j_{l-1}(\widetilde{\sigma}iR) - \frac{l+1}{\widetilde{\sigma}iR} j_l(\widetilde{\sigma}iR).$$

In view of the asymptotic behavior (A.13) of the spherical Bessel functions j_l, follows

$$2\widetilde{\sigma}ij_l'(\widetilde{\sigma}iR) + j_l(\widetilde{\sigma}iR) = \left(1 - \frac{2(l+1)}{R} \right) j_l(\widetilde{\sigma}iR) + 2\widetilde{\sigma}ij_{l-1}(\widetilde{\sigma}iR)$$

$$= \left[\left(1 - \frac{2(l+1)}{R} \right) \frac{(\widetilde{\sigma}iR)^l}{1 \cdot 3 \cdots (2l+1)} + 2\widetilde{\sigma}i \frac{(\widetilde{\sigma}iR)^{l-1}}{1 \cdot 3 \cdots (2l-1)} \right] \left(1 + O(l^{-1}) \right)$$

$$= \left[\frac{(\widetilde{\sigma}iR)^l}{1 \cdot 3 \cdots (2l+1)} + 2\widetilde{\sigma}i \frac{l}{2l+1} \frac{(\widetilde{\sigma}iR)^{l-1}}{1 \cdot 3 \cdots (2l-1)} \right] \left(1 + O(l^{-1}) \right)$$

$$= \widetilde{\sigma}i \frac{(\widetilde{\sigma}iR)^{l-1}}{1 \cdot 3 \cdots (2l-1)} \left(1 + O(l^{-1}) \right).$$

Consequently, the term in parentheses in (D.12) satisfies

$$\left(\frac{2\widetilde{\sigma}ih_l^{(1)\prime}(\widetilde{\sigma}iR) + h_l^{(1)}(\widetilde{\sigma}iR)}{2\widetilde{\sigma}ij_l'(\widetilde{\sigma}iR) + j_l(\widetilde{\sigma}iR)} j_l(\widetilde{\sigma}iR) - h_l^{(1)}(\widetilde{\sigma}iR) \right)$$

$$= \frac{2}{\widetilde{\sigma}R} \left(\frac{(\widetilde{\sigma}iR)^l}{1 \cdot 3 \cdots (2l-1)} \left(1 + O(l^{-1}) \right) \right)^{-1} \quad \text{as } l \to \infty.$$
(D.13)

The next step consists of analyzing the asymptotic behavior of the factor β_l in (D.12). Using the definition of the spherical Bessel functions, see (A.11), and the integral formula 11.2(4) in [**Luk62**], we obtain for β_l the representation

$$
\begin{aligned}
\beta_l^2 &= \int_0^R j_l(\widetilde{\sigma}ir)^2 r^2 \, \mathrm{d}r \\
&= \frac{\pi}{2\widetilde{\sigma}i} \int_0^R J_{l+\frac{1}{2}}(\widetilde{\sigma}ir)^2 r \, \mathrm{d}r \\
&= \frac{\pi}{2\widetilde{\sigma}i} \frac{R^2}{2} \left(J_{l+\frac{1}{2}}(\widetilde{\sigma}iR)^2 - J_{l+\frac{3}{2}}(\widetilde{\sigma}iR) J_{l-\frac{1}{2}}(\widetilde{\sigma}iR) \right) \\
&= \frac{R^3}{2} \left(j_l(\widetilde{\sigma}iR)^2 - j_{l+1}(\widetilde{\sigma}iR) j_{l-1}(\widetilde{\sigma}iR) \right).
\end{aligned}
$$

The asymptotic behavior (A.13) of the spherical Bessel function leads to

$$
\begin{aligned}
\beta_l^2 &= \frac{R^3}{2} \frac{1}{2l+1} \left(\frac{1}{2l+1} - \frac{1}{2l+3} \right) \left(\frac{(\widetilde{\sigma}iR)^l}{1 \cdot 3 \cdots (2l-1)} \left(1 + O(l^{-1})\right) \right)^2 \\
&= \frac{R^3}{2l+3} \left(\frac{(\widetilde{\sigma}iR)^l}{1 \cdot 3 \cdots (2l+1)} \left(1 + O(l^{-1})\right) \right)^2 \quad \text{as } l \to \infty. \qquad \text{(D.14)}
\end{aligned}
$$

Combining the estimates (D.13) and (D.14), we conclude that the singular values ς_l have the asymptotic behavior (D.11). $\qquad\square$

An immediate consequence of the previous theorem is the fact that the DA-based BLT problem, at least in the considered special case, is ill-posed of order $3/2$. We point out that this is exactly the order the operator A smoothes in Sobolev scale, provided the coefficients D, σ_a and the boundary ∂X are smooth. More precisely, for $q \in L^2(X)$ we have $Aq \in H^{3/2}(\partial X)$ and $A^* Aq \in H^3(X)$, see [**Hac92**] for instance.

Excursus: Domain Derivative of the SPECT Forward Operator

In this section we present an interesting consequence of the observations made in Subsection 2.2.1 and Subsection 4.1.1. More precisely, we derive the domain derivative of the SPECT forward operator, which coincides with the BLT forward operator in purely absorbing media, about connected domains in two dimensions rigorously. To our knowledge this has not been performed before. We are only aware of the article [**KRR11**], where the shape derivative of the least square functional involving the attenuated Radon transform is calculated. Moreover, our result developed in Theorem 6.13 holds only for ball-shaped sources.

Let us assume in this excursus that $X \subset \mathbb{R}^2$ is convex with $0 \in X$ and that X is contained in the unit ball $B_1(0)$. Latter is no restriction, since we may scale X to fit this condition.

In Subsection 2.2.1 we introduced the attenuated ray transform

$$P_{\sigma_t} q(y, \omega) = \int_{\mathbb{R}} \exp\left(- \int_t^\infty \sigma_t(y + s\omega) \, \mathrm{d}s \right) q(y + t\omega) \, \mathrm{d}t$$

for $(y, \omega) \in T = \{(x, \theta) \in \mathbb{R}^2 \times S^1 : x \in \theta^\perp\}$. The operator

$$Q \colon \mathcal{L} \to \widetilde{H}^{-1}(X), \quad Q(G) = \lambda \chi_G$$

is defined in (4.3). The aim of this excursus is to calculate the domain derivative of the operator $P_{\sigma_t} \circ Q$.

In order to do this, we have to adapt the definition of the operator Q to fit our needs. We recall that $\mathcal{S}$ is the set of subdomains of X with C^2

boundary. Let $\varepsilon > 0$ be arbitrary small. The dual space of $H^{1/2+\varepsilon}(X)$ is denoted by $\widetilde{H}^{-1/2-\varepsilon}(X)$. Now, we redefine the operator Q as

$$Q: \mathcal{S} \to \widetilde{H}^{-\frac{1}{2}-\varepsilon}(X), \quad Q(G) = \lambda \chi_G.$$

In a first step, we determine the domain derivative of Q about a connected domain $\Gamma \in \mathcal{S}$. To this end, let $h \in C_0^1(X)$ and Γ_h be the perturbation of Γ by h. Since equation (4.6) is also true for test functions $v \in H^{1/2+\varepsilon}(X)$, only the trace of v on $\partial\Gamma$ must exists[1], we have the estimate

$$\|Q(\Gamma_h) - Q(\Gamma) - \lambda h_\nu \delta_{\partial\Gamma}\|_{\widetilde{H}^{-1/2-\varepsilon}} = o(\|h\|_{C^1}),$$

which is the analog to (4.7). Consequently, the domain derivative of Q about Γ in direction h is given by

$$Q'(\Gamma)h = \lambda h_\nu \delta_{\partial\Gamma}. \tag{E.1}$$

In the next step, we show that the operator P_{σ_t} is a bounded operator from $\widetilde{H}^{-1/2-\varepsilon}(X)$ to $H^{-\varepsilon}(T)$, which is specified below. This statement directly implies the domain differentiability of the SPECT forward operator

$$P_{\sigma_t} \circ Q: \mathcal{S} \to H^{-\varepsilon}(T).$$

To obtain the continuity, we use a link to the attenuated Radon transform. As mentioned in Subsection 2.2.1, the attenuated ray transform P_{σ_t} coincides with the attenuated Radon transform in two dimensions up to notation, which is given by

$$R_{\sigma_t}q(s,\theta) = \int_{\mathbb{R}} \exp\left(-\int_t^\infty \sigma_t(s\theta + \tau\theta_\perp)\,\mathrm{d}\tau\right) q(s\theta + t\theta_\perp)\,\mathrm{d}t$$

for $(s,\theta) \in Z := \{(t,\omega) \in \mathbb{R} \times S^1\}$, where $\theta_\perp \cdot \theta = 0$ and $\det(\theta,\theta_\perp) = 1$. As in [**Nat01b**] we define the norms

$$\|g\|_{H^r(T)}^2 = \int_{S^1} \int_{\omega^\perp} \left(1 + |\eta|^2\right)^r \left|\widehat{g}(\eta,\omega)\right|^2 \mathrm{d}\eta\,\mathrm{d}\omega,$$

$$\|g\|_{H^r(Z)}^2 = \int_{S^1} \int_{\mathbb{R}} \left(1 + \xi^2\right)^r \left|\widehat{g}(\xi,\theta)\right|^2 \mathrm{d}\xi\,\mathrm{d}\theta$$

for $r \in \mathbb{R}$ and for functions g on T and Z, respectively. Herein, the Fourier transforms are understood with respect to the first variable. Easy calculations show

$$\|P_{\sigma_t}q\|_{H^r(T)} = \|R_{\sigma_t}q\|_{H^r(Z)}. \tag{E.2}$$

---

[1]This is the reason why we have to introduce the small number $\varepsilon > 0$. There is no continuous trace operator from $H^{1/2}(X)$ to $L^2(\partial\Gamma)$, since $H^{1/2}(\Gamma) = H_0^{1/2}(\Gamma)$ [**McL00**].

We need to introduce some more Hilbert spaces: Let $\mathcal{S}'(\mathbb{R}^2)$ be the space of tempered distributions, i.e., the dual space of the Schwartz space, and let the norm $\|\cdot\|_{H^r(\mathbb{R}^2)}$ be given by

$$\|v\|_{H^r(\mathbb{R}^2)} = \left(\int_{\mathbb{R}^2} \left(1 + |\xi|^2\right)^r |\hat{v}(\xi)|^2 \, d\xi \right)^{\frac{1}{2}}$$

for $v \in \mathcal{S}'(\mathbb{R}^2)$ and with $\hat{v}$ denoting the Fourier transform of v. We define the Hilbert spaces

$$H^r(\mathbb{R}^2) = \left\{ v \in \mathcal{S}'(\mathbb{R}^2) \colon \|v\|_{H^r(\mathbb{R}^2)} < \infty \right\}$$

and

$$H^r_M = \left\{ v \in H^r(\mathbb{R}^2) \colon \operatorname{supp} v \subset M \right\}$$

for a closed subset $M \subset \mathbb{R}^2$. See [**McL00, Tri78**] for more details on these spaces. From [**McL00**, Theorem 3.29] we know that

$$H^{-\frac{1}{2}-\varepsilon}_{\overline{X}} = \widetilde{H}^{-\frac{1}{2}-\varepsilon}(X).$$

This obviously implies

$$\widetilde{H}^{-\frac{1}{2}-\varepsilon}(X) \subset H^{-\frac{1}{2}-\varepsilon}_{\overline{B_1(0)}}. \tag{E.3}$$

In [**Hei86**] the following smoothing property of the two-dimensional Radon transform is shown:

$$\|R_{\sigma_t} q\|_{H^{-\varepsilon}(Z)} \leq \|q\|_{H^{-1/2-\varepsilon}(\mathbb{R}^2)} \tag{E.4}$$

for all $q \in C_0^\infty\bigl(B_1(0)\bigr)$. In view of the density of $C_0^\infty\bigl(B_1(0)\bigr)$ in $H^{-1/2-\varepsilon}_{\overline{B_1(0)}}$, cf. [**Tri78**, Theorem 1 in Section 4.3.2], the smoothing property holds for all $q \in H^{-1/2-\varepsilon}_{\overline{B_1(0)}}$. Recalling the equation (E.2), the inclusion (E.3) and the estimate (E.4), we obtain the continuity of the attenuated ray transform between $\widetilde{H}^{-1/2-\varepsilon}(X)$ and $H^{-\varepsilon}(T)$, that is,

$$\|P_{\sigma_t} q\|_{H^{-\varepsilon}(T)} \leq \|q\|_{\widetilde{H}^{-1/2-\varepsilon}}$$

for all $q \in \widetilde{H}^{-1/2-\varepsilon}(X)$.

Combining the last observation with the identity (E.1), we finally find: For $d = 2$ and for every $\varepsilon > 0$ the SPECT forward operator

$$P_{\sigma_t} \circ Q \colon \mathcal{S} \to H^{-\varepsilon}(T)$$

is differentiable and its domain derivative about the connected domain Γ in direction h is given by

$$(P_{\sigma_t} \circ Q)'(\Gamma)h = \lambda P_{\sigma_t}(h_\nu \delta_{\partial\Gamma}).$$

If, in addition, Γ is convex, then we can further specify the domain derivative by means of Remark 6.5. For $(y, \omega) \in T$, let $p_1(y, \omega) = y + \tau_1(y, \omega)\omega$ and $p_2(y, \omega) = y + \tau_2(y, \omega)\omega$ be the intersection points of the line $\{y + t\omega \colon t \in \mathbb{R}\}$ with the domain Γ such that $\omega \cdot \nu\big(p_1(y, \omega)\big) < 0$ and $\omega \cdot \nu\big(p_2(y, \omega)\big) > 0$, respectively.[2] Then, we have in view of Remark 6.5:

$$\big((P_{\sigma_t} \circ Q)'(\Gamma)h\big)(y, \omega) = \lambda \int_{\mathbb{R}} \exp\left(-\int_t^{\infty} \sigma_t(y + s\omega)\,\mathrm{d}s\right) \frac{h_\nu(y + t\omega)}{\omega \cdot \nu(y + t\omega)}$$
$$\Big(\delta\big(t - \tau_2(y, \omega)\big) - \delta\big(t - \tau_1(y, \omega)\big)\Big)\,\mathrm{d}t\,,$$

where δ is the one-dimensional delta distribution. Though this identity is essentially the same as the one in Remark 6.14, it holds for arbitrary convex domains and in a different space.

This result might be generalized to the case $d = 3$, but this is beyond the scope of this excursus. The crucial point is the smoothing property in (E.4), which has to be extended to the attenuated ray transform in higher dimensions. Though we refer in Subsection 2.2.1 to a smoothing result in three dimensions given in [SU12], this only holds for Sobolev spaces of non-negative order. Alternatively, one could try to obtain the domain derivative in case $d = 3$ by interpreting the three dimensional attenuated ray transform as family of two dimensional attenuated ray transforms as in [AK95].

---

[2] This is a similar construction as in Section 6.2.1.

List of Symbols

A	linear BLT forward operator, page 29
α	regularization parameter, page 31
$d \in \{2,3\}$	spatial dimension, page 9
D	diffusion coefficient, page 15
$\mathrm{diam}(X)$	diameter of the domain X, page 20
$\partial_{\mp}(X \times \Omega)$	inflow and outflow part of the boundary $\partial X \times \Omega$, resp., page 11
$\partial X_{\omega,\mp}$	points $x \in \partial X$ such that $\nu(x) \cdot \omega \lessgtr 0$, page 18
E_{σ_t}	attenuation function in the integral operators $\mathcal{P}$ and $\mathcal{K}$, page 92
η	scattering kernel, page 10
F	nonlinear BLT forward operator, page 30
G	geometric variable, page 30
$\mathcal{G}$	admissible set of C^2 shapes, page 38
$\gamma_{\pm}$	trace operator defined via $\gamma_{\pm}v = v\vert_{\partial_{\pm}(X \times \Omega)}$, page 18
$\mathrm{H}_{\partial\Gamma}$	additive curvature of $\partial\Gamma$, page 40
$H_{l,m}$	complex-valued spherical harmonic of degree l (and order m) for $d = 3$, page 148
$h_n^{(1)}$	spherical Hankel function of the first kind of order n, page 151
$\widetilde{H}^{-1}(X)$	dual space of $H^1(X)$, page 25
I_ν	modified Bessel functions of the first kind of order ν, page 151
J_α	Tikhonov like functional, page 31
j_n	spherical Bessel function of order n, page 151
$\mathcal{K}$	integral operator $\mathcal{K} = \mathcal{P} \circ S$, page 20

K_ν	modified Bessel functions of the second kind of order ν, page 151
$\mathcal{L}$	admissible set of measurable shapes, page 30
$\mathcal{L}(\mathcal{U}, \mathcal{V})$	space of all linear bounded operators between the Banach space $\mathcal{U}$ and $\mathcal{V}$, page 39
Λ	admissible interval for the intensity variable λ, page 30
λ	intensity variable, page 30
$\mathcal{N}(A)$	null space of the operator A, page 25
ν	outer unit normal, page 11
$\Omega = S^{d-1}$	$(d-1)$-dimensional unit sphere, page 10
$\Omega_{x,\pm}$	sets of directions pointing inward and outward the domain X, resp., page 12
$\mathcal{P}$	solution operator of the radiative transfer equation without scattering, page 20
P_l	Legendre polynomial of degree l, page 145
P_l^m	associated Legendre function of degree l and order m, page 146
P_σ	attenuated ray transform, page 22
$\mathrm{Per}(G)$	perimeter of the shape G, page 31
$\Psi'(f; h)$	(one-sided) Hadamard directional derivative of Ψ about f in direction h, page 116
$\mathcal{R}(A)$	range of the operator A, page 21
S	scattering operator, page 12
σ_a	absorption coefficient, page 10
σ_s	scattering coefficient, page 10
σ_s'	reduced scattering coefficient, page 15
σ_t	total attenuation coefficient, page 11
$\tau_\pm$	time of travel, page 18
$\mathrm{Vol}(M)$	volume or (surface) area of set or manifold M, page 13
$W_-^p(X \times \Omega)$	space of L^p functions v having a directional derivative $\omega \cdot \nabla v$ in L^p and vanishing inflow boundary values, page 18
$X \subset \mathbb{R}^d$	spatial domain, page 9
$\mathcal{Y}$	image space of BLT forward operator, page 29
$y_l^\mathrm{c}, y_l^\mathrm{s}$	spherical harmonics of degree l for $d = 2$ aka trigonometric polynomials of degree l, page 147
$Y_{l,m}$	real-valued spherical harmonics of degree l (and order m) for $d = 3$, page 148

Bibliography

[ABM06]   Hedy Attouch, Giuseppe Buttazzo, and Gérard Michaille, *Variational Analysis in Sobolev and BV Space*, MPS-SIAM Series on Optimization, Society for Industrial and Applied Mathematics, Philadelphia, 2006.

[AE84]   Jean-Pierre Aubin and Ivar Ekeland, *Applied Nonlinear Analysis*, Pure and Applied Mathematics, John Wiley & Sons, New York, 1984.

[AF03]   Robert A. Adams and John J. F. Fournier, *Sobolev spaces*, 2nd ed., Pure and Applied Mathematics, vol. 140, Elsevier/Academic Press, Amsterdam, 2003.

[Ago98]   Valeri Agoshkov, *Boundary Value Problems for Transport Equations*, Modeling and Simulation in Science, Engineering and Technology, Birkhäuser, Boston, 1998.

[AH05]   Kendall Atkinson and Weimin Han, *Theoretical Numerical Analysis*, 2nd ed., Texts in Applied Mathematics, vol. 39, Springer, New York, 2005.

[AH12]   _____, *Spherical Harmonics and Approximations on the Unit Sphere: An Introduction*, Lecture Notes in Mathematics, vol. 2044, Springer, Berlin, 2012.

[AK95]   Valentina Aguilar and Peter Kuchment, *Range conditions for the multidimensional exponential x-ray transform*, Inverse Problems **11** (1995), no. 5, 977–982.

[Arr02]   Simon R. Arridge, *Diffusion Tomography in Dense Media*, Scattering: Scattering and Inverse Scattering in Pure and Applied Science (Roy Pike and Pierre Sabatier, eds.), Academic Press, San Diego, 2002, pp. 920–933.

[AS72]   Milton Abramowitz and Irene A. Stegun (eds.), *Handbook of Mathematical Functions*, Dover, New York, 1972.

[AS09]   Simon R. Arridge and John C. Schotland, *Optical tomography: forward and inverse problems*, Inverse Problems **25** (2009), no. 12, 123010.

[AS12]   Simon R. Arridge and Otmar Scherzer, *Imaging from coupled physics*, Inverse Problems **28** (2012), no. 8, 080201.

[Bal09]   Guillaume Bal, *Inverse transport theory and applications*, Inverse Problems **25** (2009), 053001.

[Bal13]   ———, *Hybrid inverse problems and internal functionals*, Inverse Problems and Applications: Inside Out II (Gunther Uhlmann, ed.), Mathematical Sciences Research Institute Publications, vol. 60, Cambridge University Press, Cambridge, 2013.

[Ban05]   Charles Bankhead, *Bioluminescent light shines on MI*, Diagnostic Imaging, March 2005, `http://www.diagnosticimaging.com/articles/bioluminescent-light-shines-mi`.

[Bea95]   Alan F. Beardon, *The Geometry of Discrete Groups*, Graduate Texts in Mathematics, vol. 91, Springer-Verlag, New York, 1995, Corrected reprint of the 1983 original.

[Ben11]   Martin Benning, *Singular Regularization of Inverse Problems: Bregman Distances and their Applications of Variational Frameworks with Singular Regularization Energies*, PhD thesis, Westfälische Wilhelms-Universität, Münster, 2011.

[BG88]   Marcel Berger and Bernard Gostiaux, *Differential Geometry: Manifolds, Curves and Surfaces*, Graduate Texts in Mathematics, vol. 115, Springer, New York, 1988.

[BGCC99]   Harrison H. Barrett, Brandon Gallas, Eric Clarkson, and Anne Clough, *Scattered radiation in nuclear medicine: A case study on the Boltzmann transport equation*, Computational Radiology and Imaging: Therapy and Diagnostics (Christoph Börgers and Frank Natterer, eds.), The IMA Volumes in Mathematics and its Applications, vol. 110, Springer, New York, 1999, pp. 71–100.

[BO05]   Martin Burger and Stanley J. Osher, *A survey on level set methods for inverse problems and optimal design*, European J. Appl. Math. **16** (2005), no. 2, 263–301.

[BS10]   Guillaume Bal and John C. Schotland, *Inverse scattering and acousto-optic imaging*, Phys. Rev. Lett. **104** (2010), 043902.

[BT07]   Guillaume Bal and Alexandru Tamasan, *Inverse source problems in transport equations*, SIAM J. Math. Anal. **39** (2007), no. 1, 57–76.

[CD12]   Fabien Caubet and Marc Dambrine, *Localization of small obstacles in stokes flow*, Inverse Problems **28** (2012), no. 10, 105007.

[CDKT13]   Fabien Caubet, Marc Dambrine, Djalil Kateb, and Chahnaz Z. Timimoun, *A Kohn-Vogelius formulation to detect an obstacle immersed in a fluid*, Inverse Probl. Imaging **7** (2013), no. 1, 123–157.

[Ces84]   Michel Cessenat, *Théorèmes de trace L^p pour des espaces de fonctions de la neutronique*, C. R. Acad. Sc. Paris, Sér I **299** (1984), 831–834 (in French).

[Ces85]   ———, *Théorèmes de trace L^p pour des espaces de fonctions de la neutronique*, C. R. Acad. Sc. Paris, Sér I **300** (1985), 89–92 (in French).

[CK98]   David Colton and Rainer Kress, *Inverse Acoustic and Electromagnetic Scattering Theory*, 2nd ed., Applied Mathematical Sciences, vol. 93, Springer, Berlin, 1998.

[CR02]   Christopher H. Contag and Brian D. Ross, *It's not just about anatomy: In vivo bioluminescence imaging as an eyepiece into biology*, Journal of Magnetic Resonance Imaging **16** (2002), no. 4, 378–387.

[CR08]   Ana Carpio and Maria Luisa Rapún, *Topological derivatives for shape reconstruction*, Inverse Problems and Imaging (Luis L. Bonilla, ed.), Lecture Notes in Mathematics, vol. 1943, Springer, Berlin, 2008, pp. 85–133.

[CR12]   Ana Carpio and Maria Luisa Rapún, *Hybrid topological derivative and gradient-based methods for electrical impedance tomography*, Inverse Problems **28** (2012), no. 9, 095010.

[CS96]   Mourad Choulli and Plamen Stefanov, *Inverse scattering and inverse boundary value problems for the linear Boltzmann equation*, Comm. Partial Differential Equations **21** (1996), no. 5-6, 763–785.

[CS99]   _____, *An inverse boundary value problem for the stationary transport equation*, Osaka J. Math. **36** (1999), 87–104.

[CWK+05] Wenxiang Cong, Ge Wang, Durairaj Kumar, Yi Liu, Ming Jiang, Lihong Wang, Eric Hoffman, Geoffrey McLennan, Paul McCray, Joseph Zabner, and Alexander Cong, *Practical reconstruction method for bioluminescence tomography*, Opt. Express **13** (2005), 6756–6771.

[CZ67]   Kenneth M. Case and Paul F. Zweifel, *Linear Transport Theory*, Addison-Wesley Series in Nuclear Engineering, Addison-Wesley, Reading, Mass., 1967.

[DCL12]   Andriano De Cezaro and Antonio Leitão, *Level-set approaches of L_2-type for recovering shape and contrast in ill-posed problems*, Inverse Probl. Sci. Eng. **20** (2012), no. 4, 571–587.

[DFN84]   Boris A. Dubrovin, Anatolij T. Fomenko, and Sergej P. Novikov, *Modern Geometry—Methods and Applications. Part I: The Geometry of Surfaces, Transformation Groups, and Fields*, Graduate Texts in Mathematics, vol. 93, Springer-Verlag, New York, 1984, Translated from the Russian by Robert G. Burns.

[DL00a]   Robert Dautray and Jacques-Louis Lions, *Mathematical Analysis and Numerical Methods for Science and Technology: Evolution Problems I*, vol. 5, Springer, Berlin, 2000.

[DL00b]   _____, *Mathematical Analysis and Numerical Methods for Science and Technology: Evolution Problems II*, vol. 6, Springer, Berlin, 2000.

[Dor98]   Oliver Dorn, *A transport-backtransport method for optical tomography*, Inverse Problems **14** (1998), no. 5, 1107–1130.

[Dor02]   _____, *Shape reconstruction in scattering media with voids using a transport model and level sets*, Can. Appl. Math. Q. **10** (2002), 239–275.

[DZ11]   Michel C. Delfour and Jean-Paul Zolésio, *Shapes and Geometries : Analysis, Differential Calculus, and Optimization*, 2nd ed., Advances in Design and Control, Society for Industrial and Applied Mathematics, Philadelphia, 2011.

[EFS10]   Herbert Egger, Manuel Freiberger, and Matthias Schlottbom, *On forward and inverse models in fluorescence diffuse optical tomography*, Inverse Probl. Imaging **4** (2010), no. 3, 411–427.

[Eic11]   Joseph A. Eichholz, *Discontinuous Galerkin Methods for the Radiative Transfer Equation and its Approximations*, PhD thesis, The University of Iowa, Iowa City, 2011.

[Eic13]   _____, *RTEPACK Manual*, version from April 05, 2013.

[Eke74]   Ivar Ekeland, *On the variational principle*, J. Math. Anal. Appl **47** (1974), 324–353.

[Eke79]   _____, *Nonconvex minimization problems*, Bull. Am. Math. Soc., New
             Ser. **1** (1979), 443–474.

[ES12]   Herbert Egger and Matthias Schlottbom, *A mixed variational framework
             for the radiative transfer equation*, Math. Models Methods Appl. Sci. **22**
             (2012), no. 03, 1150014.

[ES13]   _____, *An L^p theory for stationary radiative transfer*, Appl. Anal. (2013),
             published online August 02, 2013.

[FGS98]   Willi Freeden, Theo Gervens, and Michael Schreiner, *Constructive Approx-
             imation on the Sphere*, Numerical Mathematics and Scientific Computa-
             tion, Oxford University Press, New York, 1998.

[GC13]   Rongfang Gong and Xiaoliang Cheng, *An optimal finite element error esti-
             mate for an inverse problem in multispectral bioluminescence tomography*,
             IMA J. Appl. Math. (2013), published online June 28, 2013.

[GCH10]   Rongfang Gong, Xiaoliang Cheng, and Weimin Han, *Bioluminescence to-
             mography for media with spatially varying refractive index*, Inverse Probl.
             Sci. Eng. **18** (2010), no. 3, 295–312.

[Giu84]   Enrico Giusti, *Minimal Surfaces and Functions of Bounded Variation*,
             Monographs in Mathematics, vol. 80, Birkhäuser, Boston, 1984.

[GLYZ08]   Wei Gong, Ruo Li, Ningning Yan, and Weibo Zhao, *An improved error
             analysis for finite element approximation of bioluminescence tomography*,
             J. Comput. Math. **26** (2008), no. 3, 297–309.

[GZ10a]   Hao Gao and Hongkai Zhao, *Multilevel bioluminescence tomography based
             on radiative transfer equation part 1: l1 regularization*, Opt. Express **18**
             (2010), no. 3, 1854–1871.

[GZ10b]   _____, *Multilevel bioluminescence tomography based on radiative trans-
             fer equation part 2: total variation and l1 data fidelity*, Opt. Express **18**
             (2010), no. 3, 2894–2912.

[GZLJ04]   Xuejun Gu, Qizhi Zhang, Lyndon Larcom, and Huabei Jiang, *Three-
             dimensional bioluminescence tomography with model-based reconstruction*,
             Opt. Express **12** (2004), no. 17, 3996–4000.

[Hac92]   Wolfgang Hackbusch, *Elliptic Differential Equations: Theory and Numer-
             ical Treatment*, Springer Series in Computational Mathematics, vol. 18,
             Springer, Berlin, 1992.

[HB09]   Martin Hanke-Bourgeois, *Grundlagen der Numerischen Mathematik und
             des Wissenschaftlichen Rechnens*, 3rd ed., Vieweg + Teubner, Wiesbaden,
             2009 (in German).

[HCKW09]   Weimin Han, Wenxiang Cong, Kamran Kazmi, and Ge Wang, *An inte-
             grated solution and analysis of bioluminescence tomography and diffuse
             optical tomography*, Comm. Numer. Methods Engrg. **25** (2009), no. 6, 639–
             656.

[HCW06a]   Weimin Han, Wenxiang Cong, and Ge Wang, *Mathematical theory and
             numerical analysis of bioluminescence tomography*, Inverse Problems **22**
             (2006), 1659–1675.

[HCW06b]   _____, *Mathematical study and numerical simulation of multispectral bi-
             oluminescence tomography*, Int. J. Biomed. Imaging **2006** (2006), Article
             ID 54390.

[HEHL11]   Weimin Han, Joseph A. Eichholz, Jianguo Huang, and Jia Lu, *RTE-based bioluminescence tomography: A theoretical study*, Inverse Probl. Sci. Eng. **19** (2011), 435–459.

[Hei86]   Uwe Heike, *Single-photon emission computed tomography by inverting the attenuated Radon transform with least-squares collocation*, Inverse Problems **2** (1986), no. 3, 307–330.

[Het99]   Frank Hettlich, *The Domain Derivative in Inverse Obstacle Problems*, Habilitation thesis, Friedrich-Alexander-Universität, Erlangen, 1999.

[HG41]   Louis G. Henyey and Jesse L. Greenstein, *Diffuse radiation in the Galaxy*, Astrophysical Journal **93** (1941), 70–83.

[HGC13]   Weimin Han, Rongfang Gong, and Xiaoliang Cheng, *A general framework for integration of bioluminescence tomography and diffuse optical tomography*, Inverse Probl. Sci. Eng. (2013), published online May 07, 2013.

[HHE10]   Weimin Han, Jianguo Huang, and Joseph A. Eichholz, *Discrete-ordinate discontinuous Galerkin methods for solving the radiative transfer equation*, SIAM J. Sci. Comput. **32** (2010), no. 2, 477–497.

[HKCW07]   Weimin Han, Kamran Kazmi, Wenxiang Cong, and Ge Wang, *Bioluminescence tomography with optimized optical parameters*, Inverse Problems **23** (2007), no. 3, 1215–1228.

[HLN12]   Michael Hintermüller, Antoine Laurain, and Antonio A. Novotny, *Second-order topological expansion for electrical impedance tomography*, Advances in Computational Mathematics **36** (2012), no. 2, 235–265.

[Hob55]   Ernest W. Hobson, *The Theory of Spherical and Ellipsoidal Harmonics*, Chelsea Publ., New York, 1955, unaltered reprint of the original ed., 1931, Cambridge University Press.

[HPUU09]   Michael Hinze, Rene Pinnau, Michael Ulbrich, and Stefan Ulbrich, *Optimization with PDE Constraints*, Mathematical Modelling: Theory and Applications, vol. 23, Springer, 2009.

[HR96]   Frank Hettlich and William Rundell, *Iterative methods for the reconstruction of an inverse potential problem*, Inverse Problems **12** (1996), 251–266.

[HSK+09]   Weimin Han, Haiou Shen, Kamran Kazmi, Wenxiang Cong, and Ge Wang, *Studies of a mathematical model for temperature-modulated bioluminescence tomography*, Appl. Anal. **88** (2009), no. 2, 193–213.

[HT11]   Helmut Harbrecht and Johannes Tausch, *An efficient numerical method for a shape-identification problem arising from the heat equation*, Inverse Problems **27** (2011), no. 6, 065013.

[HW07]   Weimin Han and Ge Wang, *Theoretical and numerical analysis on multispectral bioluminescence tomography*, IMA J. Appl. Math. **72** (2007), no. 1, 67–85.

[HW08]   ———, *Bioluminescence tomography: biomedical background, mathematical theory, and numerical approximation*, J. Comput. Math. **26** (2008), no. 3, 324–335.

[Hyv07]   Nuutti Hyvönen, *Fréchet derivative with respect to the shape of a strongly convex nonscattering region in optical tomography*, Inverse Problems **23** (2007), 2249–2270.

[IK08]   Kazufumi Ito and Karl Kunisch, *Lagrange Multiplier Approach to Variational Problems and Applications*, Advances in Design and Control, vol. 15, Society for Industrial and Applied Mathematics, Philadelphia, 2008.

[IK10]   Olha Ivanyshyn and Rainer Kress, *Identification of sound-soft 3D obstacles from phaseless data*, Inverse Probl. Imaging **4** (2010), no. 1, 131–149.

[Isa06]   Victor Isakov, *Inverse Problems for Partial Differential Equations*, 2nd ed., Applied Mathematical Sciences, vol. 127, Springer, New York, 2006.

[JW08]   Ming Jiang and Ge Wang, *Uniqueness results for multi-spectral bioluminescence tomography*, Mathematical Methods in Biomedical Imaging and Intensity-Modulated Radiation Therapy (IMRT) (Yair Censor, Ming Jiang, and Alfred K. Louis, eds.), CRM Series, vol. 7, Edizioni della Normale, Pisa, 2008, pp. 153–172.

[Kel99]   Carl T. Kelley, *Iterative Methods for Optimization*, Frontiers in Applied Mathematics, vol. 18, Society for Industrial and Applied Mathematics, Philadelphia, 1999.

[Kir93]   Andreas Kirsch, *The domain derivative and two applications in inverse scattering theory*, Inverse Problems **9** (1993), no. 1, 81–96.

[Kir11]   Andreas Kirsch, *An Introduction to the Mathematical Theory of Inverse Problems*, 2nd ed., Applied Mathematical Sciences, vol. 120, Springer, New York, 2011.

[Klo09]   Alexander D. Klose, *Radiative transfer of luminescence light in biological tissue*, Light Scattering Reviews 4 (Alexander A. Kokhanovsky, ed.), Springer Praxis Books, Springer, Berlin, 2009, pp. 293–345.

[KNH05]   Alexander D. Klose, Vasilis Ntziachristos, and Andreas H. Hielscher, *The inverse source problem based on the radiative transfer equation in optical molecular imaging*, J. Comput. Phys. **202** (2005), no. 1, 323–345.

[KR12]   Tim Kreutzmann and Andreas Rieder, *Geometric reconstruction in bioluminescence tomography*, IWRMM Preprint **12** (2012), no. 6, to appear in Inverse Probl. Imaging.

[Kre89]   Rainer Kress, *Linear Integral Equations*, Applied Mathematical Sciences, vol. 82, Springer-Verlag, Berlin, 1989.

[Kre08]   Tim Kreutzmann, *Biolumineszenz-Tomographie: Theorie und Rekonstruktionsalgorithmen*, Diplomarbeit, Universität Karlsruhe (TH), Karlsruhe, 2008, (in German).

[KRR11]   Esther Klann, Ronny Ramlau, and Wolfgang Ring, *A Mumford-Shah level-set approach for the inversion and segmentation of SPECT/CT data*, Inverse Probl. Imaging **5** (2011), no. 1, 137–166.

[Kun01]   Leonid A. Kunyansky, *A new SPECT reconstruction algorithm based on the Novikov explicit inversion formula*, Inverse Problems **17** (2001), no. 2, 293–306.

[Lan93]   Serge Lang, *Real and Functional Analysis*, 3rd ed., Graduate Texts in Mathematics, vol. 142, Springer, New York, 1993.

[Leb73]   Nikolaj N. Lebedew, *Spezielle Funktionen und ihre Anwendung*, Bibliogr. Inst., Mannheim, 1973 (in German).

[LHFS13]   Antoine Laurain, Michael Hintermüller, Manuel Freiberger, and Hermann Scharfetter, *Topological sensitivity analysis in fluorescence optical tomography*, Inverse Problems **29** (2013), no. 2, 025003.

[LM84]   Elmer E. Lewis and Warren F. Miller, *Computational Methods of Neutron Transport*, Wiley, New York, 1984.

[LS03]   Antonio Leitão and Otmar Scherzer, *On the relation between constraint regularization, level sets, and shape optimization*, Inverse Problems **19** (2003), L1–L11, Corrigendum in Inverse Problems **22** (2006), 1507.

[Luk62]   Yudell L. Luke, *Integrals of Bessel Function*, McGraw-Hill, New York, 1962.

[LZD⁺09]   Yujie Lu, Xiaoqun Zhang, Ali Douraghy, David Stout, Jie Tian, Tony F. Chan, and Arion F. Chatziioannou, *Source reconstruction for spectrally-resolved bioluminescence tomography with sparse a priori information*, Opt. Express **17** (2009), no. 10, 8062–8080.

[McL00]   William C. McLean, *Strongly Elliptic Systems and Boundary Integral Equations*, Cambridge University Press, Cambridge, 2000.

[MK97]   Mustapha Mokhtar-Kharroubi, *Mathematical Topics in Neutron Transport Theory : New Aspects*, Series on Advances in Mathematics for Applied Sciences, vol. 46, World Scientific, Singapore, 1997.

[MS89]   David Mumford and Jayant Shah, *Optimal approximations by piecewise smooth functions and associated variational problems*, Comm. Pure Appl. Math. **42** (1989), no. 5, 577–685.

[Nat01a]   Frank Natterer, *Inversion of the attenuated Radon transform*, Inverse Problems **17** (2001), no. 1, 113–119.

[Nat01b]   Frank Natterer, *The Mathematics of Computerized Tomography*, Classics in Applied Mathematics, vol. 32, Society for Industrial and Applied Mathematics, Philadelphia, 2001.

[NFTP03]   Antonio A. Novotny, Raúl A. Feijóo, Edgardo Taroco, and Claudio Padra, *Topological sensitivity analysis*, Comput. Meth. Appl. Mech. Engrg. **192** (2003), no. 7–8, 803–829.

[Nov02]   Roman G. Novikov, *An inversion formula for the attenuated X-ray transformation*, Arkiv för Matematik **40** (2002), no. 1, 145–167.

[NRWW05]   Vasilis Ntziachristos, Jorge Ripoll, Lihong V. Wang, and Ralph Weissleder, *Looking and listening to light: the evolution of whole-body photonic imaging*, Nat. Biotech. **23** (2005), no. 3, 313–320.

[NW01]   Frank Natterer and Frank Wübbeling, *Mathematical methods in image reconstruction*, SIAM Monographs on Mathematical Modeling and Computation, Society for Industrial and Applied Mathematics, Philadelphia, 2001.

[NW06]   Jorge Nocedal and Stephen J. Wright, *Numerical Optimization*, 2nd ed., Springer Series in Operations Research and Financial Engineering, Springer, New York, 2006.

[Rie03]   Andreas Rieder, *Keine Probleme mit Inversen Problemen*, Vieweg, Wiesbaden, 2003 (in German).

[RR04]   Michael Renardy and Robert C. Rogers, *An Introduction to Partial Differential Equations*, 2nd ed., Texts in Applied Mathematics, vol. 13, Springer, New York, 2004.

[RR07]   Ronny Ramlau and Wolfgang Ring, *A Mumford-Shah level-set approach for the inversion and segmentation of X-ray tomography data*, J. Comput. Phys. **221** (2007), 539–557.

[RR10]   ———, *Regularization of ill-posed Mumford-Shah models with perimeter penalization*, Inverse Problems **26** (2010), 115001.

[San96]   Fadil Santosa, *A level-set approach for inverse problems involving obstacles*, ESAIM, Control Optim. Calc. Var. **1** (1996), 17–33.

[Set99]   James A. Sethian, *Level Set Methods and Fast Marching Methods*, 2nd ed., Cambridge Monographs on Applied and Computational Mathematics, vol. 3, Cambridge University Press, Cambridge, 1999.

[Sha90]   Alexander Shapiro, *On concepts of directional differentiability*, J. Optim. Theory Appl. **66** (1990), no. 3, 477–487.

[Sim80]   Jacques Simon, *Differentiation with respect to the domain in boundary value problems*, Numer. Funct. Anal. Optim. **2** (1980), 649–687.

[SU08]   Plamen Stefanov and Gunther Uhlmann, *An inverse source problem in optical molecular imaging*, Anal. PDE **1** (2008), no. 1, 115–126.

[SU12]   Plamen Stefanov and Gunther Uhlmann, *The geodesic X-ray transform with fold caustics*, Anal. PDE **5** (2012), no. 2, 219–260.

[SZ92]   Jan Sokolowski and Jean-Paul Zolésio, *Introduction to Shape Optimization: Shape Sensitivity Analysis*, Springer Series in Computational Mathematics, vol. 16, Springer, Berlin, 1992.

[Tao12]   Terence Tao, *Topics in Random Matrix Theory*, Graduate Studies in Mathematics, vol. 132, American Mathematical Society, Providence, RI, 2012.

[TC05]   Steve H. Thorne and Christopher H. Contag, *Using in vivo bioluminescence imaging to shed light on cancer biology*, Proceedings of the IEEE **93** (2005), no. 4, 750–762.

[Tri78]   Hans Triebel, *Interpolation Theory, Function Spaces, Differential Operators*, North-Holland Mathematical Library, vol. 18, North-Holland Publishing Co., Amsterdam, 1978.

[Wat52]   George N. Watson, *A Treatise on the Theory of Bessel Functions*, 2nd ed., University Press, Cambridge, 1952.

[WCD$^+$06]   Ge Wang, Wenxiang Cong, Kumar Durairaj, Xin Qian, Haiou Shen, Patrick Sinn, Eric Hoffman, Geoffrey McLennan, and Michael Henry, *In vivo mouse studies with bioluminescence tomography*, Opt. Express **14** (2006), no. 17, 7801–7809.

[WCL$^+$06]   Ge Wang, Wenxiang Cong, Yi Li, Weimin Han, Durai Kumar, Xin Qian, Haiou Shen, Ming Jiang, Tie Zhou, Jiantao Cheng, Jie Tian, Yujie Lv, Hui Li, and Jie Luo, *Recent development in bioluminescence tomography*, 3rd IEEE International Symposium on Biomedical Imaging: Nano to Macro, 2006, pp. 678–681.

[Wer07]   Dirk Werner, *Funktionalanalysis*, 6th ed., Springer-Lehrbuch, Springer, Berlin, 2007 (in German).

[Wey39]   Hermann Weyl, *On the volume of tubes*, Amer. J. Math. **61** (1939), 461–472.

[WG89]   Zhu Xi Wang and Dun Ren Guo, *Special Functions*, World Scientific, Singapore, 1989.

[WHM]   Ge Wang, Eric Hoffman, and Geoffrey McLennan, *Systems and methods for bioluminescencent computed tomographic reconstruction*, US Patent Number 8,090,431, US provisional patent application filed in March 2003, US patent application filed in March 2004.

[WLJ04]   Ge Wang, Yi Li, and Ming Jiang, *Uniqueness theorems in bioluminescence tomography*, Medical Physics **31** (2004), 2289–2299, Erratum in Medical Physics **32** (2005), 3059.

[Wlo87]   Joseph Wloka, *Partial Differential Equations*, Cambridge University Press, Cambridge, 1987.

[WN03]   Ralph Weissleder and Vasilis Ntziachristos, *Shedding light onto live molecular targets*, Nat. Med. **9** (2003), no. 1, 123–128.

[ZLC12]   Xiaoqun Zhang, Yujie Lu, and Tony Chan, *A novel sparsity reconstruction method from Poisson data for 3D bioluminescence tomography*, J. Sci. Comput. **50** (2012), no. 3, 519–535.